AF228882

Eating Disorders

ON THE RISE

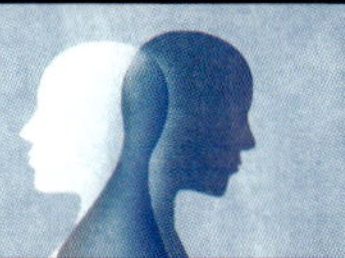

Don Nardo

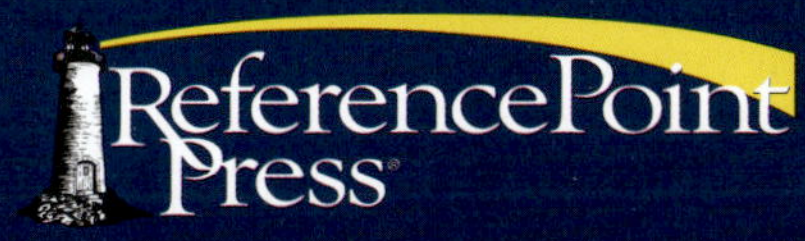

ReferencePoint
Press

San Diego, CA

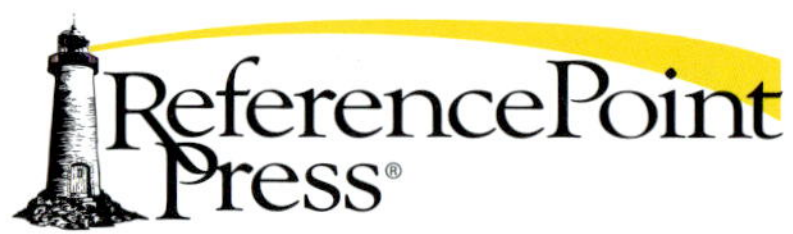

© 2023 ReferencePoint Press, Inc.
Printed in the United States

For more information, contact:
ReferencePoint Press, Inc.
PO Box 27779
San Diego, CA 92198
www.ReferencePointPress.com

Picture Credits:

Cover: SpeedKingz/Shutterstock.com
 7: Tinseltown/Shutterstock.com
10: Motortion/iStock
13: SB Arts Media/Shutterstock.com
17: indira's work/Shutterstock.com
22: miodrag ignjatovic/iStock
25: KatarzynaBialasiewicz/iStock
29: Motortion Films/Shuttestock.com
33: Maury Aaseng
36: SpeedKing/Shutterstock.com
38: Juice Dash/Shutterstock.com
45: Prostock-studio/Shutterstock.com
49: SMEEitz/Shutterstock.com
53: Elena Valebnaya/Shutterstock.com

LIBRARY OF CONGRESS CATALOGING-IN-PUBLICATION DATA

Names: Nardo, Don, 1947- author.
Title: Eating disorders on the rise / by Don Nardo.
Description: San Diego, CA : ReferencePoint Press, 2023. | Series: Mental
  health crisis | Includes bibliographical references and index.
Identifiers: LCCN 2021062867 (print) | LCCN 2021062868 (ebook) | ISBN
  9781678202781 (library binding) | ISBN 9781678202798 (ebook)
Subjects: LCSH: Eating disorders.
Classification: LCC RC552.E18 N372 2023 (print) | LCC RC552.E18 (ebook) |
  DDC 616.85/26--dc23/eng/20220112
LC record available at https://lccn.loc.gov/2021062867
LC ebook record available at https://lccn.loc.gov/2021062868

CONTENTS

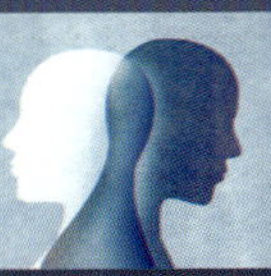

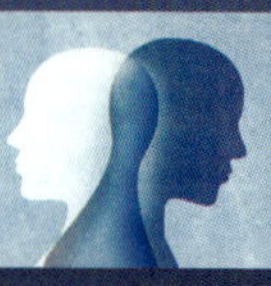

A Significant Social and Medical Hazard

Now in her midtwenties, Sara looks back at her high school years and wishes she could have talked herself out of a course of action that would have serious consequences for her health and well-being. Back then, she says, she was an awkward teenager "with braces, glasses, acne, and a sweet, yet painfully shy, personality."[1] Because she was a bit chubby, she adds, she was also self-conscious about her weight.

Sara's body-image concerns unexpectedly came into play one day after school when she was watching a TV talk show. The subject was eating disorders, and one of the guests, a teenage girl, described how she regularly overate and then rid herself of the food by vomiting. At that moment, Sara recalls, "A light went off in my head. I made my way to the washroom in a daze. I looked at myself in the mirror, still not entirely sure what I was doing. Then I pulled my hair back into a ponytail, knelt over the toilet and made myself sick. I wish, with all my heart, that I could tell every young girl or boy who is contemplating that very action for the first time . . . not to."[2]

Eliminating food that way—which medical experts call purging—may seem like a convenient, largely harmless way to control one's weight. But the reality, Sara states with a surety that comes from personal experience, is that "it wreaks havoc on your body. [You] may think you'll only do it once in a while, but like any addiction it will become your life. I wish I could tell [people] to say NO to that first, not so powerful, urge, to get out while they still can."[3]

An Alarming Number of Cases

The condition that both Sara and the girl she saw on TV suffer from is called bulimia nervosa (or simply "bulimia"), and it is one of the three primary eating disorders. The other two are anorexia nervosa ("anorexia" for short) and binge-eating disorder. These conditions are far more widespread than most people realize, since those who have them represent all ages, genders, and economic and social classes.

The sheer number of sufferers is alarming. According to the National Eating Disorders Association (NEDA), these conditions affect some 20 million women and 10 million men in the United States alone, or nearly one-tenth of the nation's population. Of the male sufferers, "we think the 10 million number is probably actually larger,"[4] says Claire Mysko, the NEDA's director. Many men, she explains, assume that only females get such disorders, and therefore those men do not realize that they themselves have one.

Mysko and other experts on eating disorders add that the number of individuals reporting these disorders increased during the COVID-19 pandemic, which began in earnest in the early months of 2020. For instance, a study reported in the *International Journal of Eating Disorders* in July 2020 found that anorexics "experienced a worsening of symptoms as the pandemic hit." Similarly, bulimics and binge eaters "reported increases in their binge-eating episodes and urges to binge."[5] In addition, the NEDA reported an increase of at least 70 percent in calls to its national help line in late 2020 and early 2021.

Multiple reasons have been cited for this ominous increase. But topping the list is the worldwide surge in anxiety and stress the pandemic brought about. In the words of Kathy Katella of the Yale School of Medicine, "The stress we've all faced during the pandemic has played out in a wide variety of ways, including weight gain for many, and for those with eating disorders—an exacerbation [worsening] of symptoms."[6]

Raising Awareness

While the pandemic has worsened the symptoms, people with eating disorders normally experience physical and emotional problems of varying seriousness and intensity. These include unhealthy weight gain or loss, poor nutrition, stress, mood swings, substance abuse, and clinical depression, to name only a few. Moreover, the most extreme cases can result in suicidal thoughts or even death. Eating disorders have therefore become a significant social and medical hazard. According to the world-famous Mayo Clinic, these conditions can "negatively impact your health, your emotions, and your ability to function in important areas of life."[7]

Leading national efforts to raise awareness of eating disorders and help sufferers are organizations like the NEDA, the National Association of Anorexia Nervosa and Associated Disorders, and the National Institute of Mental Health (NIMH). But increasingly, such awareness has also come from celebrities with the courage to come forward and describe their personal struggles with these

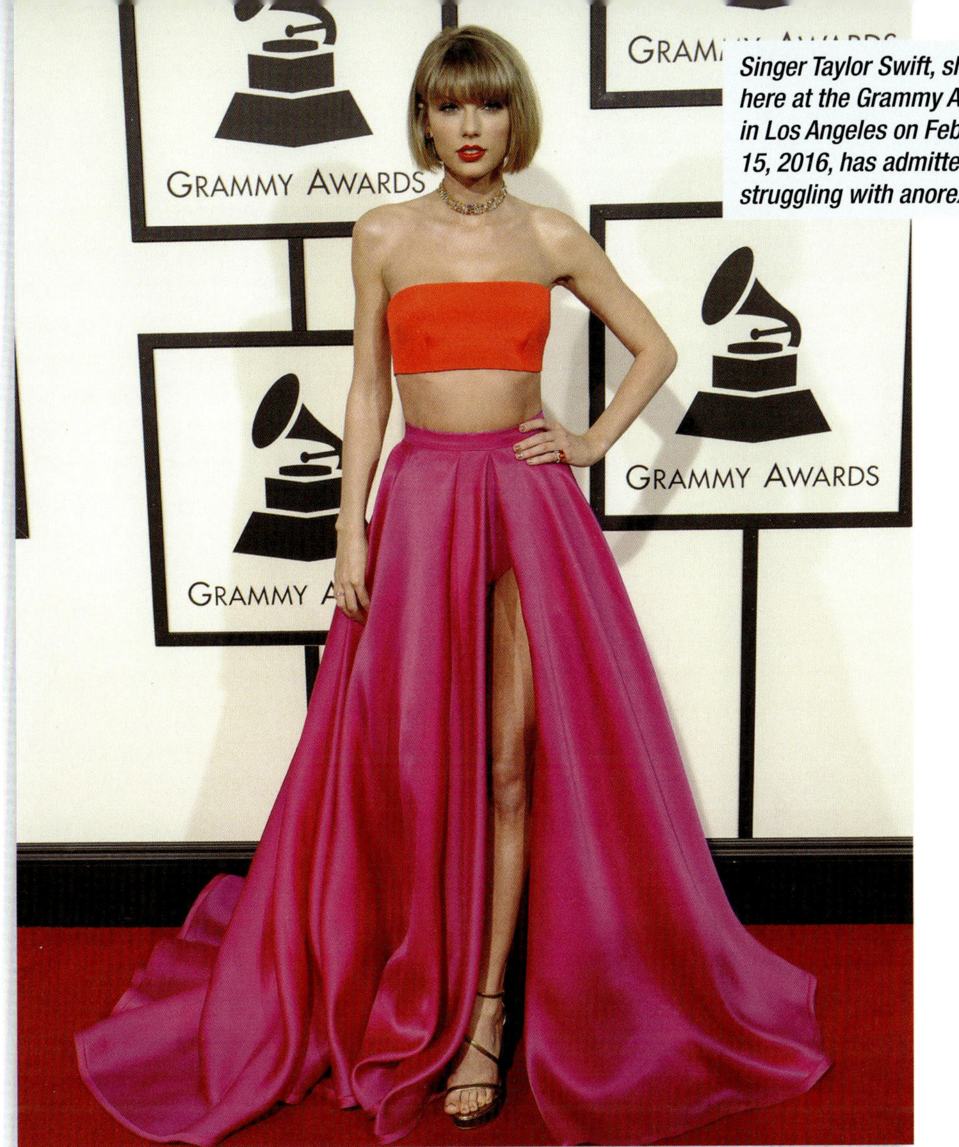

Singer Taylor Swift, shown here at the Grammy Awards in Los Angeles on February 15, 2016, has admitted to struggling with anorexia.

conditions. One of the most recent examples was popular singer Taylor Swift, who in 2020 revealed her own battle with anorexia. Film director Lana Wilson, who made a documentary about Swift, says, "I think it's really brave to see someone who is a role model for so many girls and women be really honest about that. I think it will have a huge impact."[8]

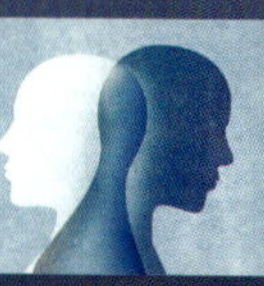

CHAPTER ONE

The Big Three Eating Disorders

"I have [been] suffering from anorexia for the past 3 years," says Ben, a thirty-year-old male business professional. "During this time it has taken a devastating toll on my physical and emotional health, and my professional and personal life." Like many young adults in their twenties, Ben took little time or interest in preparing healthy food. As a result, he explains, "my weight had crept up gradually over the years." Then suddenly, his relationship with his girlfriend ended. He says she "explicitly told me that she was no longer attracted to me due to my weight."[9]

At that point, Ben says, his life began to undergo a major change for the worse. The stress from the breakup steadily took a toll, and he found himself gradually eating less food and losing weight. As time went on, he became so absorbed in this behavior that he bought a scale and began weighing himself several times a day.

"From there," Ben continues, "my life degenerated extremely rapidly. Food started dominating my thoughts and feelings. Losing weight became an obsession, a very dangerous one." As the months dragged on, he progressively ate less and less while exercising more and more. "Nothing was left to chance," he remembers. "My weight had dropped further. I was so focused on my weight loss that I didn't even realize how my life was falling apart. Being overweight was all that I had known, and having now lost a large number of [pounds], I would literally do anything to jealously protect the weight loss I had achieved. Eating now dominated every part of my life."[10]

Closely Related Conditions

Eating disorders, including the one Ben developed—anorexia—are medical conditions in which the sufferers develop unhealthy, potentially dangerous eating habits and patterns. In most cases the people in question consume either too little or too much food and end up experiencing diverse physical, emotional, and at times social problems. Some of these include depression, abuse of laxatives and other drugs, self-loathing and unhappiness, insomnia or sleep apnea, muscle or joint pain, diabetes, and heart disease. In addition, the most serious cases can result in hospitalization or death. Indeed, these conditions "are not a fad, phase or lifestyle choice," states an NEDA spokesperson. They are "potentially life-threatening conditions that affect a person's emotional and physical health."[11]

Medical experts recognize several different eating disorders. However, some are rare, and three—sometimes called "the big three"—are by far the most common and widespread; they are binge eating, bulimia, and anorexia. Each has recognizable symptoms that differentiate it from the other two. Nevertheless, the three are closely related. That is, they are all physical responses to people's misuse of food. Therefore, binge eaters, bulimics, and anorexics often display some of the same symptoms and behaviors.

Moreover, it is not unusual for one of the three eating disorders to lead to another. For example, bulimics almost always start out as binge eaters. And many anorexics initially go through binge-eating and bulimic stages.

Regular Bouts of Major Overeating

Binge eating (which has been called compulsive overeating and other names in the past) can be a sort of gateway to the usually more detrimental bulimia and anorexia. Binge eating is certainly the most prevalent of the three disorders. According to the NEDA and other expert sources, in the United States roughly 3.5 percent of adult women and 2 percent of adult men are binge eaters. That translates into some 11.5 million women and 6.6 million men.

Typically, a binge eater habitually devours enormous amounts of food in a single sitting. Often, favorite bingeing items include highly caloric ones such as cake, pie, doughnuts, ice cream, pizza, and potato chips. "I had a love-hate relationship with food," says former binge eater Rachel Goodman. "As soon as I took a bite of a 'forbidden food' (hello, cheesecake and ice cream!), it

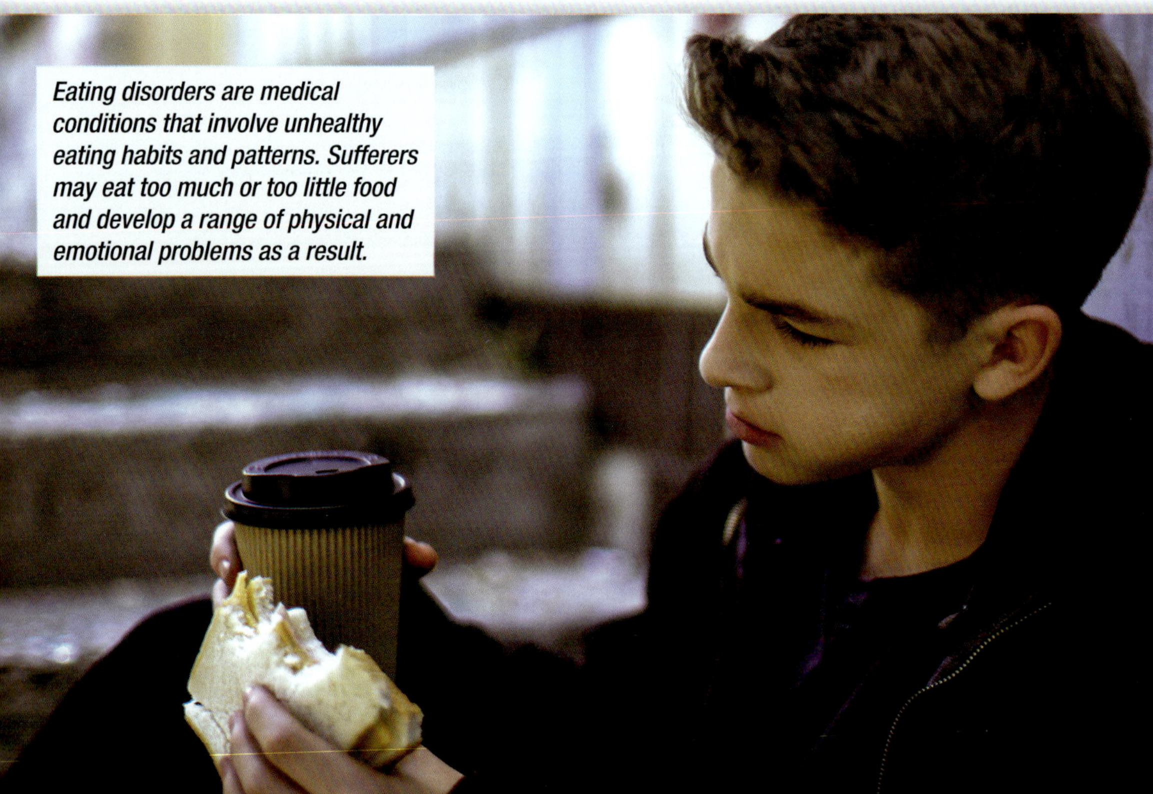

Eating disorders are medical conditions that involve unhealthy eating habits and patterns. Sufferers may eat too much or too little food and develop a range of physical and emotional problems as a result.

[wasn't] long before I said 'to hell with it' and went to town on all the things I was going to keep off limits tomorrow."[12] In spite of this common approach, however, it is not unusual for binge eaters to sometimes consume large portions of *healthy* foods like vegetables, fruits, and chicken.

The frequency of such splurges tends to vary from person to person. Some binge eaters do so about once a week or even once every two weeks. Others binge several times a week. What is more certain is that binge eaters usually become overweight to one degree or another. Desiring to shed the extra pounds, they may quit bingeing for a few weeks or a month or two. In most cases, though, they will eventually return to a pattern of regular bouts of major overeating.

Symptoms of Bulimia

Many binge eaters continue to have such episodes of food abuse for years and in some cases for the rest of their lives. However, some of them end up moving on to the second of the big three eating disorders—bulimia—characterized by purging the food consumed in a binge. An office worker named Jack resorted to that approach. He remembers a binge in which he eagerly stuffed down large numbers of pastries in only a few minutes and his extreme reaction to doing so. "I felt sick," he says, "queasy, guilty. I started to panic. Literally, [I felt] as though I was having a panic attack. I ran to the toilets and got rid of it all."[13]

Jack was revolted by that incident and did not want to repeat it. But he soon found that it was difficult to fight the urges he felt. He recalls:

Eventually I would give in and binge which would always lead to a purge. Over time it became stronger and more frequent. I began to wonder if there was something deeply wrong with me. I wondered why I couldn't be normal around food. I was constantly exhausted, stressed and moody. I would pretend to everyone to be this happy-go-lucky guy, but deep down I was . . . miserable, scared, [and] confused.[14]

The NEDA, Eating Disorder Hope, and other similar organizations estimate that most bulimics binge and purge once or more per week. A few sufferers do so almost every day. They often feel shame and therefore try to hide their condition from family and friends. However, extreme cases of the condition are hard to hide. As Eating Disorder Hope points out, a bulimic tends to display certain telltale symptoms, "many of which are the direct result of self-induced vomiting or other forms of purging, especially if the binge/purge cycle is repeated several times a week and/or day."[15]

Among the revealing symptoms of bulimia is regularly using the bathroom after a meal. Others include frequently smelling like vomit, having enlarged glands in the neck area (caused by repeated vomiting), and regular fluctuations in a person's weight. At times, a person's binges will cause weight gain. In contrast, after repeated vomiting episodes, that individual will sometimes experience weight loss.

A Powerful Fear of Becoming Fat

In a few cases bulimics' weight losses will steadily outnumber and in time totally replace their periods of weight gain. These individuals may then become anorexic. Often the most physically damaging of the big three eating disorders, anorexia is characterized by a powerful fear of becoming fat, and the sufferer typically severely reduces her or his food intake, sometimes to the point of self-starvation. According to the NIMH:

People with anorexia nervosa typically weigh themselves repeatedly, severely restrict the amount of food they eat, often exercise excessively, and/or may force themselves to vomit or use laxatives to lose weight. Anorexia nervosa has the highest mortality rate of any mental disorder. While many people with this disorder die from complications associated with starvation, others die of suicide.[16]

The NIMH goes on to list common symptoms of anorexia, including extreme thinness and a persistent quest to become thinner. Also typical is a distorted body image, in which individuals see themselves as chubby even when they are abnormally thin. Other symptoms that frequently appear over time are muscle wasting and weakness, thinning of the bones, and brittle hair and nails. The lack of foods can also produce severe constipation, excessive

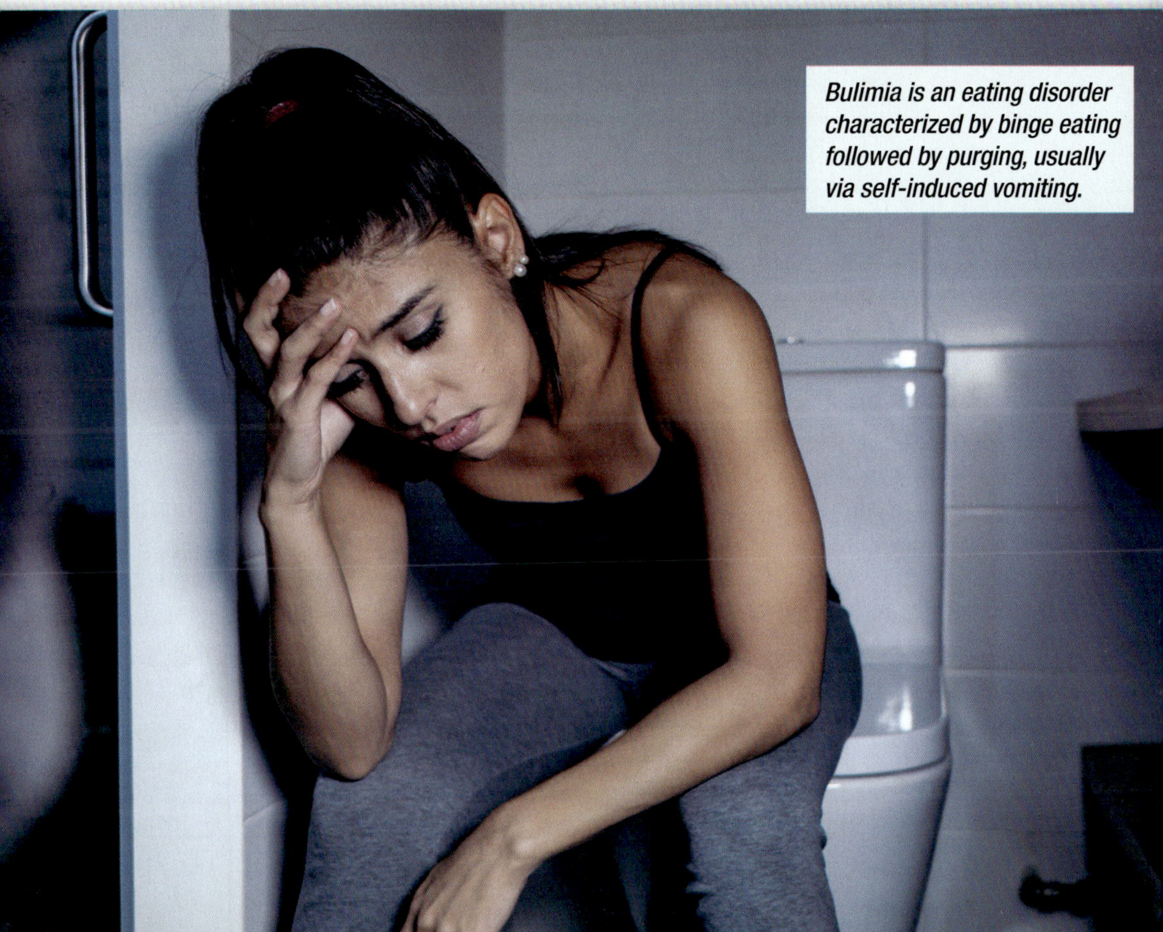

Bulimia is an eating disorder characterized by binge eating followed by purging, usually via self-induced vomiting.

tiredness, and low blood pressure. In the most extreme cases, the sufferer may develop heart problems, brain damage, or multiple organ failure, followed by death.

Experts point out that every case of anorexia is somewhat different. So not all sufferers display every symptom. What all sufferers do experience, however, is emotional distress and at times feelings of hopelessness, fear, and agony. Amanda Goheen, who developed anorexia at age twelve, recalls:

> Throughout my adolescence years I struggled with depression [and] low self-esteem. . . . I turned to self-injury as well as a way to cope. I began to spiral downward both emotionally and physically in my early 20's. I was hospitalized many times for depression, suicide, and mood issues. When I was 22, I was at a severely low weight, weak and emotionally unstable. I was told I would not see my 23rd birthday.[17]

Another young woman who suffered from anorexia—Julie Saunders—was also wracked by feelings of hopelessness and the dread of possibly dying at a young age. "I cried when I thought of food and berated myself for eating," she remembers. "I was a shell of who I once was. Every day I thought to myself that I couldn't live this way forever, but the alternative was me gaining weight, and at the time, that was even worse than being consumed by the monster inside me that was my eating disorder."[18]

What Causes Eating Disorders?

Goheen, Saunders, and the others naturally wanted to know what caused their eating disorders because knowing that might allow them to overcome those debilitating conditions. The answers they sought were elusive, however. Unfortunately for sufferers, the root causes of eating disorders are complex and still not fully identified. The staff of *Psychology Today* explains that

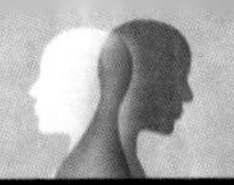

Now in her twenties, Chani Coady says she was overweight in her early school years, and that made her the object of frequent ridicule. She tried losing weight, but the diets she went on did not work, and she ended up becoming psychologically reliant on food—which she often ate in secret. "I have been on every diet I can think of," she states.

> I'd lose weight for a little bit, but it always came back. The most extreme weight loss came with a doctor-supervised diet where I ate almost nothing. The weight fell off, and my hair fell out. My nails were breaking. I was constantly cold and tired. I was miserable and I realized that I was slowly killing myself. My body was starved. Every time I saw food, I needed to eat it; I became obsessed with finding and eating food. I ate secretly. I ate not-so-secretly. I would panic every time I needed to eat in front of someone. I eventually became so out of control that I came full circle: I came to the realization that I was slowly killing myself with food.

Chani Coady, "I Just Am," *Stories of Hope* (blog), National Eating Disorders Association, 2021. www.nationaleatingdisorders.org.

these conditions have no single cause. More significantly, the staff adds, "it's not yet understood why ostensibly voluntary behaviors associated with eating turn into disorders for some people but not for others."[19]

Nevertheless, doctors and other experts do recognize that certain individual physical, medical, emotional, and social factors often contribute to the onset of eating disorders. One such factor appears to be biological and chemical in origin. The *Psychology Today* staffers say that "appetite control and the regulation of food intake is highly complex, with many hormones in the brain and the body signaling hunger and satiety [the feeling of fullness]."[20] Varying mixes of these chemicals apparently can make some people more likely than others to develop an eating disorder.

Some other factors that contribute to eating disorders are more psychological or emotional in nature. Low self-esteem, for example, may make some individuals more likely to indulge in abusive behavior, including food abuse. That is what happened to Ben when he was in his twenties. His self-esteem was so low that he saw himself as an unworthy person and was also extremely unhappy with his weight and how he looked. He recalls:

> Having been overweight for most of my life, I always dreamed about being fit, toned, muscular, and attractive. In my late teens I made a conscious effort to lose weight, and simultaneously hit the gym. . . . I was proud of my efforts to reach a healthy weight, but was increasingly concerned about putting weight back on. . . . Eventually I started to make myself vomit after some meals if I felt that I had overdone it.[21]

Perfectionism and Depression

Unhappiness with one's personal appearance can also lead to the self-imposed pursuit of perfection. In turn, that might lead a person to eat either less or more in order to create a "more per-fect" body. This is what a young man named Seth Bland went through. As he tells it:

> My eating disorder behaviors were always geared towards being perfect. Perfectionism is a terrible personality trait, bar none one of the worst out there. Mine just happened to gain a face through an eating disorder. I would con-stantly beat myself up for falling short at school, sports, faith, family life, etc. to the point that I just gave up. I quit playing sports, I quit on God, I lashed out at my family, ignored them every possible moment, and my friends be-came distant and nothing to me.[22]

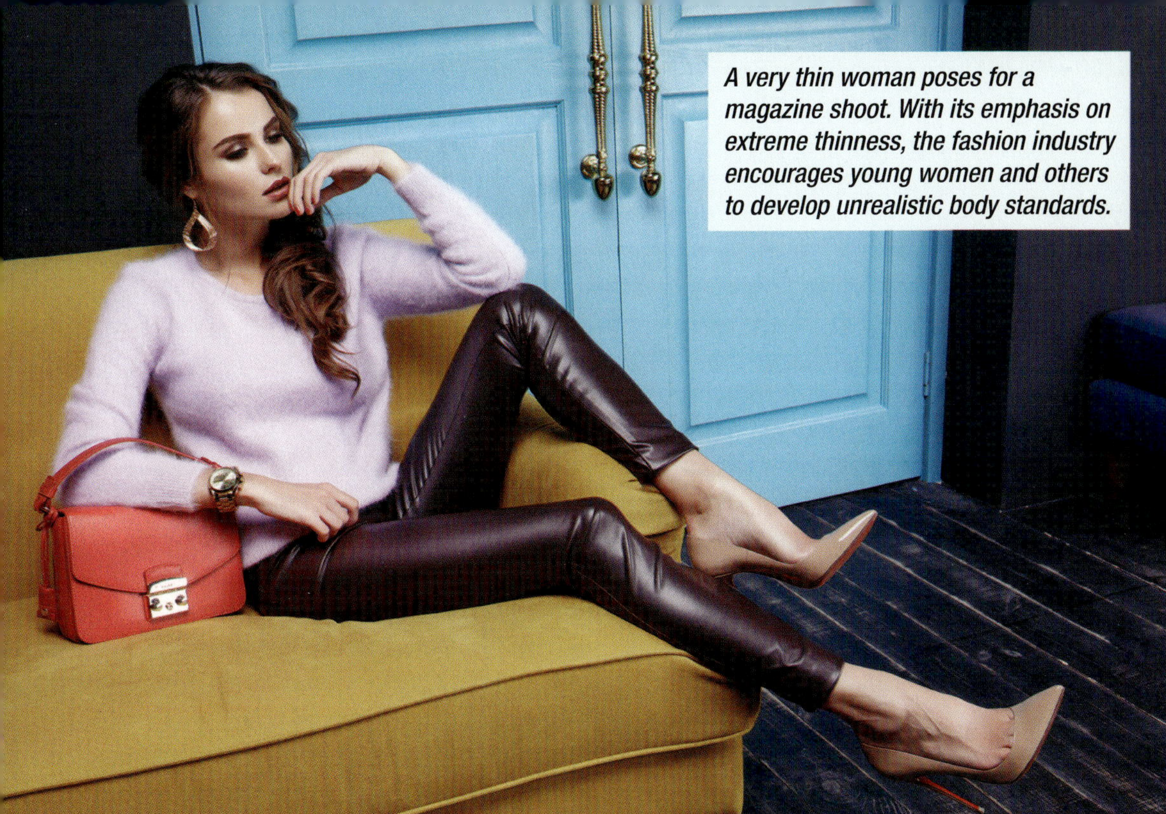

A very thin woman poses for a magazine shoot. With its emphasis on extreme thinness, the fashion industry encourages young women and others to develop unrealistic body standards.

Other emotional factors that contribute to developing eating disorders include excessive amounts of stress in people's lives as well as clinical depression. The latter is a state of mind in which people feel not only sad or gloomy but also hopeless, and it is not unusual for sufferers to see life as no longer worth living. People who feel that despondent might turn to abusing food because they reason that there is nothing to lose, since death will likely come soon anyway. Furthermore, the eating disorder itself almost always ends up deepening the state of that depression. This was what happened to Saunders, who later admitted, "I was seconds away from giving up. An eating disorder is a slow death, a[n] unspoken suicide."[23]

Factors such as low self-esteem, perfectionism, and depression can be and often are reinforced by social images and trends depicted in the media.

> "An eating disorder is a slow death, a[n] unspoken suicide."[23]
>
> —Julie Saunders, a woman who suffers from anorexia

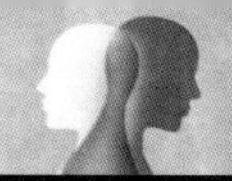

Although binge eating, bulimia, and anorexia are the most prevalent eating disorders, medical science does recognize other, much less common ones. One, orthorexia, is characterized by a strong, even obsessive, emphasis on "pure" or "clean" eating—that is, consuming foods that are as completely natural and unprocessed as possible. Because experts still know relatively little about this condition, they are unable to estimate the number of sufferers with any degree of accuracy. Another rare food-related condition is rumination disorder. Those who have it repeatedly regurgitate food after eating it and hold it in the mouth for a while. They then either spit it out or re-swallow it. Still another uncommon and little understood eating problem is known as avoidant/restrictive food intake disorder. People who suffer from it consume less food than they should each day, but not because of fear of gaining weight. Rather, these individuals may eat less out of a lack of interest in food. In particular, they avoid foods having certain physical qualities, such as a specific color, texture, taste, or smell. Or these persons may avoid food out of a fear of choking.

Particularly damaging is the strong emphasis on thinness that appears in print ads for clothes, in movies, and on TV and the internet. Especially targeted in these venues are young women, who may try to imitate excessively skinny models and actresses.

Far from Hopeless

Ben's and Bland's struggles with their weight in their adult years is regularly echoed in the millions of both men and women who have gone on various types of reducing diets. Medical experts point out that most of the fad diets promoted in magazines and on TV and the internet ultimately fail. Not only do most dieters gain back the lost pounds, they also sometimes develop urges to binge on fattening foods. And of those who become habitual binge eaters, some go on to suffer from bulimia or anorexia. Eating Disorder Hope warns, "Jumping on the bandwagon of popular diet fads can also be a gateway to eating disorder habits and behaviors."[24]

In whatever way or ways that various people acquire eating disorders, sufferers invariably endure a difficult, uncomfortable ordeal. Yet the situation is far from hopeless. Several effective treatments exist. As recovered bulimic Ashley Marcin puts it, "If you're dealing with an eating disorder, I encourage you to seek help. . . . You can do it today. Don't let yourself live with an eating disorder for another week, month, or year. . . . Don't make my mistake and fill your memory book with reminders of your eating disorder instead of the truly important moments in your life."[25]

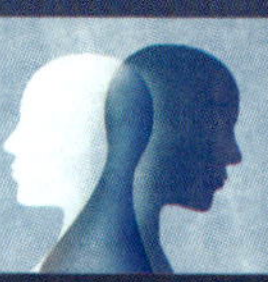

CHAPTER TWO

The COVID-19 Pandemic and the Rise in Eating Disorders

The COVID-19 pandemic changed California-born Jane's life in ways that she could not have imagined when the news of the disease first appeared. Partway through her sophomore year at college, the school closed temporarily, and she traveled home for a hiatus of unknown length. There she found conditions starkly different from those in the busy academic and social schedule she was used to. "All of a sudden," she recalls, "I had nothing going on."[26]

With so much free time on her hands, Jane decided to take advantage of the situation and get into top physical condition. At college she had not had enough time for regular exercise, and now she had ample time for it. She also decided to try, in her words, to "eat in a very concerted and controlled and deliberate way." That ended up translating into eating a good deal less than she normally did, in hopes that it would help her trim off some unwanted pounds. Eventually, however, she realized that she was consuming "an insufficient amount for my body. I masqueraded under some false notion that it was fine and I was fine, and became honestly so hungry I didn't know I was hungry and didn't know that over the course of a year I had lost much of my personality and ability to feel."[27]

At the end of that year, Jane finally went to her family doctor. His diagnosis was that she had developed an eating disorder, more specifically anorexia nervosa. It was unfortunate, he told her, that thanks indirectly to the pandemic, she now faced many months of learning to reregulate and regain control of her eating habits.

Meanwhile, college junior Ruby Samim had a different experience involving the pandemic and food. She was already a binge eater when COVID-19 appeared, so her months in quarantine did not prompt her eating disorder. However, certain factors during that period made her condition worse. "I felt like I was spending a lot of time on social media and TikTok," she explains. And most of that time she felt compelled to compare her body to those of online "celebrities and influencers."[28] That induced her to starve herself in between binges, and she found herself fighting the urge to vomit after she did overeat. She now advises friends to reduce their exposure to social media in order to avoid negative influences that might affect their eating habits.

An Upsurge in Eating Disorder Cases

Jane and Samim were not alone in their adverse food-related reactions to the societal turmoil brought about by the COVID-19 pandemic. Only a few months into the lockdowns and quarantines enacted across the United States, doctors and medical researchers began seeing a tangible nationwide increase in new cases of eating disorders and a worsening of existing cases. A survey funded by the NIMH in July 2020, for example, showed that 60 percent of the anorexics interviewed felt that their physical and emotional conditions had worsened during the pandemic's initial few months. Likewise, 30 percent of the bulimics and binge eaters surveyed reported similar setbacks.

Moreover, half a year later, in January 2021 the NEDA announced that demand for its online and phone services had increased more than 40 percent during 2020. In addition, "eating disorder diagnoses increased 15 percent in 2020 among people under 30 compared to previous years," say University of Virginia medical experts Julia F. Taylor and Sara Groff Stephens. Percentages of people over thirty were up as well. "We are a physician and a psychotherapist who specialize in treating eating disorders [and] we've seen the increased demand for eating disorder services in our own clinic."[29]

Similar clinics across the country that treat eating disorders have witnessed the same steep rise in demand for help. The case of Kirsty Batten, now twenty-five, was one of the new ones, as she was diagnosed with symptoms of bulimia a few months after the pandemic began. Having had friends over the years who had struggled with eating disorders, she was fully aware of how debilitating such conditions could be and admits to experiencing "a sense of impending doom"[30] after her diagnosis.

As for those individuals who already had bulimia or one of the other eating disorders when the pandemic first struck, typical was

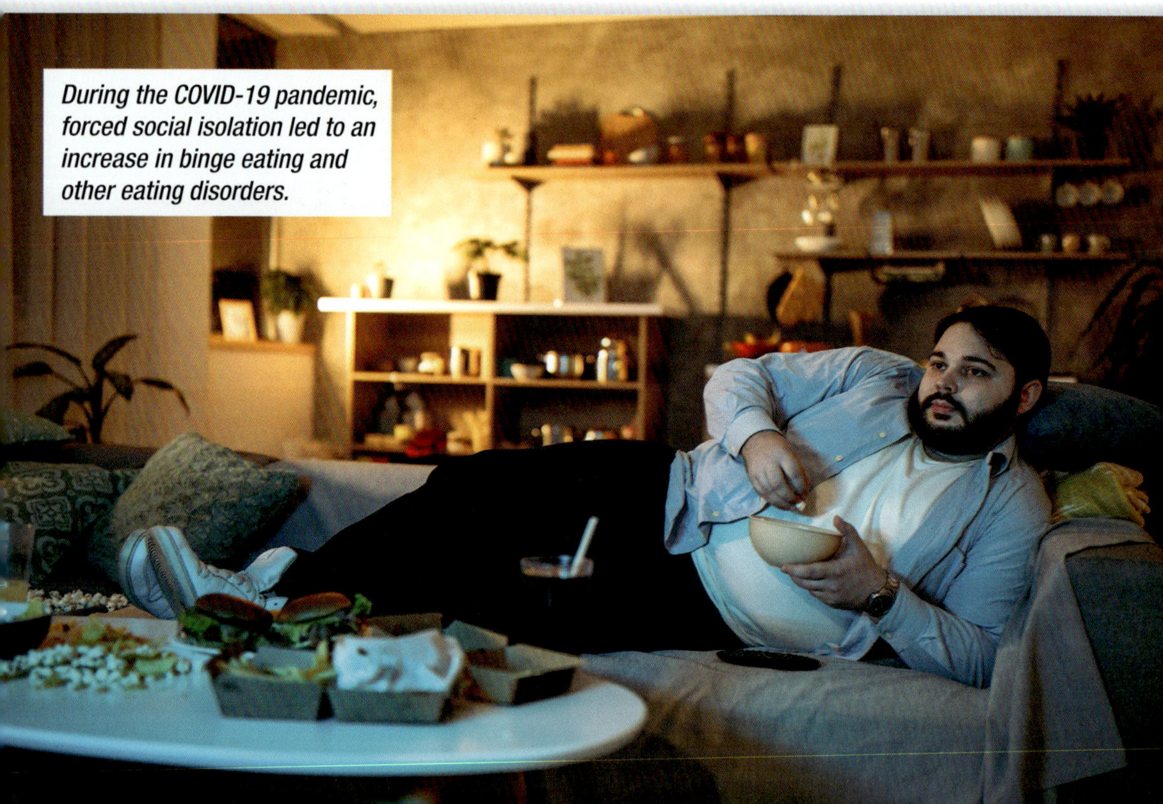

During the COVID-19 pandemic, forced social isolation led to an increase in binge eating and other eating disorders.

what twenty-two-year-old Lucy Fetterman experienced. She had been diagnosed with anorexia well before the COVID-19 onslaught started. It had taken her a couple of years to seriously come to grips with her disorder, she remembers, until one day when she looked at her reflection in a mirror and

said to herself, "Is this how I want to spend my 20s? Is this how I want to go through the rest of my life? I saw myself choosing my eating disorder and disordered activities over my friends and family." Not long after learning to largely manage her eating habits, however, the pandemic struck, and Fetterman found her normal life routines disrupted as never before. "Not only eating, but all of my habits kind of shifted,"[31] she says. In faithfully practicing social distancing, she often found herself alone and with little to do. As a result, once again she struggled hard to control her food-related urges.

Loss of Social Support and Isolation

Fetterman was one of many Americans of all ages who experienced both major changes in their normal life routines and isolation brought about by the frequent social distancing that was a hallmark of the pandemic. Jane, from California, also felt the effects of altered daily routines and isolation, as did large numbers of people across the country. And not surprisingly, these were among the leading ways that the pandemic stimulated an increased occurrence of eating disorders.

Looking first at the forced changes in daily routines brought on by staying home more often, experts say that this reduced people's access to social support. That is, a person with an eating disorder or who is prone to developing one had less interaction with family and friends. That included people who normally gave the person sound advice on various matters or who were usually available to help the person during a crisis. The pandemic therefore disrupted the social support network of untold numbers

Eating Disorders Often Go Untreated in Men

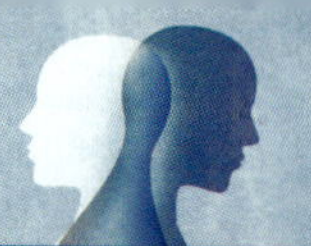

Medical journalist Jennifer Clopton made the following comments about eating disorders in men in an article on that topic for the popular medical website WebMD.

> Historically, and socially, these disorders are most commonly thought of as affecting women. But research shows not only that they happen regardless of gender, but also that they are likely underrepresented, under-diagnosed, and under-treated in men. The National Eating Disorders Association says 10 million males will be affected in their lifetimes. Men make up 15% of cases, including anorexia nervosa, bulimia nervosa, and binge-eating disorder, recent research shows. [Also], 22% of young men turn to dangerous means to bulk up muscle with disordered eating behaviors. Men with anorexia nervosa may face harsher stigmatization from their peers or go undiagnosed because of the stereotype that anorexia nervosa is a "female" disorder." . . . A [2019] study highlights the stigma, shame, and isolation men often have that may impede and delay treatment. . . . [In addition, says Lauren Smolar, director of programs at the NEDA], "because of stigma and stereotypes, males often have a harder time being diagnosed and receiving treatment for an eating disorder."

Jennifer Clopton, "Men's Eating Disorders Often Not Recognized," WebMD, September 6, 2019. www.webmd.com.

of people. And that made some of those people feel a perceived loss of control over their lives. In turn, that feeling of lost control made it more likely for them either to develop an eating disorder or have an existing disorder get worse.

For some individuals, that loss of personal support worked in tandem with increased isolation from society in general. A study conducted in 2020 in the United Kingdom and published in the *Journal of Eating Disorders* found that, of 129 people with eating disorders interviewed, 86 percent experienced major feelings of social isolation during the pandemic. For many of those same people, most of whom ranged in age from their twenties to their sixties, the isolation they endured was a major hinderance. According to the study, this was because those individuals felt that "spending time with friends and family represents a vital factor in their eating disorder recovery."[32]

Real-life examples of the negative effects of this sort of isolation were common during the pandemic. Ryan Sheldon, a model in Los Angeles who is a binge eater, says, "Eating disorders are isolating to begin with, and here we are, isolating ourselves even more."[33] Similarly, New York City resident Stephanie Parker describes how being confined to her studio apartment for months on end aggravated the symptoms of her anorexia: "The OCD [obsessive-compulsive disorder] and anxiety [I experienced from being shut away so long] just made my eating disorder more intense, and for me that meant I would become obsessed with cleaning everything and then checking in with myself to see if I deserved to eat."[34]

—New York City resident Stephanie Parker

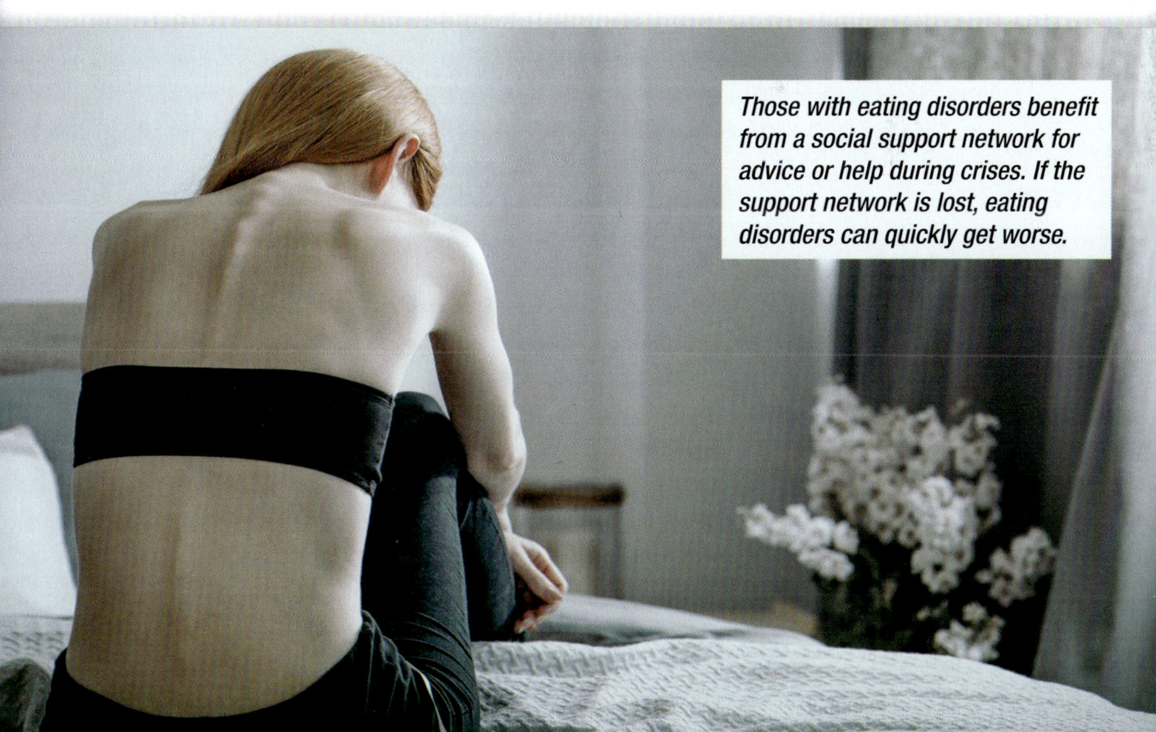

Those with eating disorders benefit from a social support network for advice or help during crises. If the support network is lost, eating disorders can quickly get worse.

Increased Stress and Anxiety

In addition to her feelings of being confined and isolated during the pandemic, Parker mentions her anxiety, or mental state of extreme worry and unease. Experts point out that the COVID-19 lockdowns unleashed feelings of anxiety that penetrated all parts of the country.

The pandemic also dished out a lot of stress, which tends to go hand in hand with or even initiate anxiety. According to the 2020 UK study in the *Journal of Eating Disorders,* "The prolonged stress of living in challenging environments [can] be particularly detrimental for those experiencing eating disorders."[35] For many people the COVID-19 lockdowns created an extremely challenging environment, one in which they primarily worried about catching the disease. But as the pandemic dragged on, people experienced rising anxiety because of breakdowns in normal routines and habits and a perceived lack of control over their lives.

All that increased stress and anxiety in turn made it far more difficult for people with eating disorders to regulate and control their eating habits. As a result, an estimated 85 percent of those individuals experienced a worsening of their symptoms. Binge eaters, for instance, tended to binge more often or to consume larger numbers of calories in each binge. Similarly, most bulimics binged and purged more often, and many anorexics ate even less food than they did before the pandemic struck.

This overall increase in incidents of food abuse among eating disorder sufferers had the general effect of making them even more anxious, paranoid, or unhappy. During the pandemic-motivated lockdown, one anorexic based in the United Kingdom lost his job and hunkered down in his parents' house. He later told one of the 2020 UK study's interviewers, "I'm trapped at home with people who don't know I have anorexia. I am hiding and lying constantly."[36]

Other interviewees complained that the people they lived with during the pandemic were often critical of their eating behaviors. As one eating disorder sufferer put it, "I have much less choice of what I eat and I have to eat most of my meals in front (and in scrutiny) of others and that is causing enormous stress."[37] Still others said they had to contend with family members who worried that if they did not eat enough they would be more likely to contract COVID-19. One anorexic stated, "My mother is particularly concerned about me because I 'do not give my body enough energy to overcome the virus' if I contracted it, and she wants me to eat more because of this. This is weighing on my mind because I absolutely do not want to do this."[38]

Men with Eating Disorders

The COVID-19 pandemic did more than exacerbate the incidence of and damage done by eating disorders. Experts point out that the social distancing and lockdowns brought about by COVID-19 also highlighted the specific social groups that these harmful conditions have often tended to target in recent years. As Taylor and Stephens maintain, eating disorders have for many years been underdiagnosed in certain sectors of the population. Two major examples are males and members of LGBTQ community. "The recent COVID-related increase in patients presenting for [medical] care," Taylor and Stephens write, "has reinforced that no group is immune from [eating disorders]."[39]

Regarding men and eating disorders, Taylor and Stephens explain, the most recent statistics indicate that one in seven of them will suffer from one of those conditions by age forty. That translates to at least 10 million adult men of varying ages. The number of men diagnosed with eating disorders rose steadily in the three decades preceding the pandemic and jumped higher still after COVID-19 struck. The exact number of male sufferers both before and during the pandemic remains undetermined. But doctors, therapists, and clinics all noticed a considerable increase in males seeking help for eating disorders after COVID-19 appeared. "I've been practicing for over 20 years," remarks Alice Baker, a certified eating disorder dietitian in Orlando, Florida, "and I've never seen such a stark increase in need."[40]

As for why so many men developed eating disorders during the pandemic, the answer appears to be twofold. On the one hand, some of them developed those conditions because of the societal disruptions that negatively affected everyone during that period. These included abrupt changes in daily routines, stress, anxiety, isolation, and loss of social support.

On the other hand, other men who either developed an eating disorder or had an existing one worsen during the COVID-19 pandemic did so as a result of factors that affect men far more often than women. According to University of California, San Francisco, professor of pediatrics Jason Nagata, "The symptoms that one thinks about for a classic eating disorder are extreme or unhealthy weight loss behaviors, like vomiting or fasting. But the idealized masculine body image is actually not [aligned] toward that same ideal. [Instead] a lot of guys are trying to get muscular and bulk up, so a lot of those weight loss behaviors don't actually apply to them."[41]

Nagata and other authorities on eating disorders say that men in their twenties and thirties, and even some older men, are significantly influenced by images of muscular males. The latter range from popular sports figures to Hollywood actors to powerful superheroes in comic books and movies. In hopes of imitating those hypermasculine role models, an unknown number of men eat either more or less than normal amounts of food and in some cases develop an eating disorder.

Eating Disorders Among LGBTQ Folk

Numerous individuals in the LGBTQ community also came down with eating disorders during the COVID-19 pandemic. Statistics show that even under normal conditions, gay, bisexual, and transgender people are more prone to developing such disorders than straight people are. According to the NEDA, for instance, "Gay

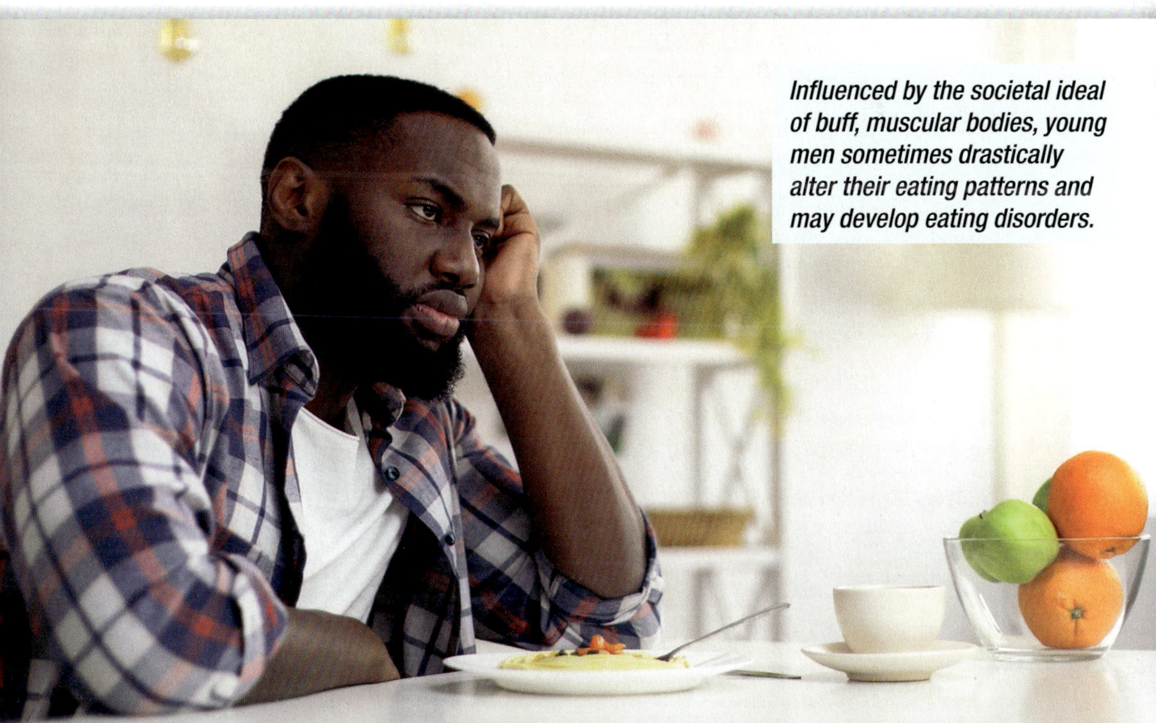

Influenced by the societal ideal of buff, muscular bodies, young men sometimes drastically alter their eating patterns and may develop eating disorders.

males are thought to only represent 5 percent of the total male population but among males who have eating disorders, 42 percent identify as gay, [and] gay males are seven times more likely to report binging and twelve times more likely to report purging than heterosexual males."[42]

The reasons for this are not yet understood. However, the NEDA and other similar organizations, along with most professional therapists, believe that the frequent bias and discrimination that LGBTQ folk endure significantly increase their stress levels and feelings of isolation. In turn, that makes them more likely to abuse food. Based on that supposition, as the pandemic commenced, some medical experts worried that the extra stress and isolation brought on by the pandemic might push many LGBTQ individuals into abusing food more often than they normally would. A study sponsored in 2021 by the National Institutes of Health concluded that "LGBTQ individuals experienced uniquely high levels of pandemic-related stress, [which] was associated with increased eating disorder symptoms and perceived weight gain. . . . [Thus] eating concerns, physical exercise constraints, and weight concerns were important to LGBTQ people's perceived health challenges during the pandemic."[43]

Thus, the COVID-19 pandemic created many and varied challenges to people who already suffered from eating disorders or were physically and/or mentally predisposed to develop one. The 2020 UK study summarized these challenges, while pointing out that hope exists to alleviate some of their negative impacts. The pandemic's adverse effects, the study concludes, are due in large part to

> changes to individuals' regular routine, living situation, time spent with friends and family, access to treatment, engagement in physical activity, relationship with food, and use of technology. The research [supporting the study] discusses how these issues can be addressed via further developments within healthcare [and government] policy. [In the future] this could benefit those experiencing eating disorders and also mental health issues more broadly.[44]

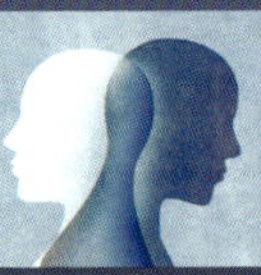

CHAPTER THREE

Eating Disorders in Teens

A few months after the COVID-19 pandemic began in early 2020, thirteen-year-old Alyssa told her parents that she strongly desired to make it onto the soccer team of her middle school. She realized that for her to be competitive in the upcoming tryouts, she had to be in the best physical condition possible. She eagerly started exercising vigorously every day. She lost a few pounds, which at first seemed logical, since she was burning a lot more calories than she usually did. But as time went on, she also tended to eat less than she normally did. So she kept shedding pounds, and soon her parents began to worry.

Eventually, Allyssa felt too weak to continue her exercise regimen, and her parents took her to the Children's SHINE (Support and Help in Nutrition and Exercise) Clinic at the Children's of Alabama hospital in Birmingham, Alabama. There the doctors diagnosed her with anorexia nervosa. At that point Alyssa became one of the growing number of teenagers who either developed an eating disorder or had an existing one worsen during the pandemic.

The medical director of the SHINE Clinic, Stephanie B. Wallace, admitted to being surprised at the large numbers of young people who were developing eating disorders in the pandemic's wake. In 2021 she remarked,

"Personally, and in our clinics, we're seeing a lot of young people who are facing all kinds of mental health disorders that are on the rise, as our young people have been in the COVID-19 pandemic for over a year, and eating disorders are included."[45]

These increases in hospitalizations due to eating disorders were confirmed by several studies completed in 2020 and 2021. One frequently cited 2020 survey was conducted by the medical journal *Epic Health*. It found that eating disorder–related hospital admissions among adolescent girls had increased by 30 percent during the pandemic.

Alarming Rates Among Adolescents

Regardless of such increases, before the pandemic adolescents were already developing eating disorders at alarming rates, rates that were consistently higher than those of adults. Thus, the fact that this trend accelerated after COVID-19's appearance made an already serious problem even worse. Indeed, according to the NIMH, just prior to the pandemic, roughly 4 to 5 percent of females aged thirteen to eighteen nationwide had an eating disorder of one kind or another. Also, about 1.5 percent of males in the country in that same age group had eating disorders. (It is impossible to translate these percentages into precise numbers, but rough estimates would be 440,000 to 550,000 adolescent females and 165,000 adolescent males.)

These general figures show that these disorders are particularly prevalent among adolescent girls. Other studies have corroborated that fact. For instance, in 2019 the widely respected *Journal of Abnormal Psychology* reported that the findings of its study published in 2010 were still valid. That earlier survey had followed the lives of a group of 496 teenage girls in a single US city for eight years. Among those young women, about the same proportion as in 2019—5 percent—had displayed symptoms of anorexia, bulimia, or binge eating.

Moreover, not only were eating disorders in adolescent girls still highly prevalent in society in 2019, the harmful effects of these

Although eating disorders can develop at any age, they are more likely to begin before the age of twenty. This is the finding of a ten-year study by the National Association of Anorexia Nervosa and Associated Disorders. That study revealed that 86 percent of individuals with an eating disorder experienced the symptoms of the disorder before they turned twenty years old.

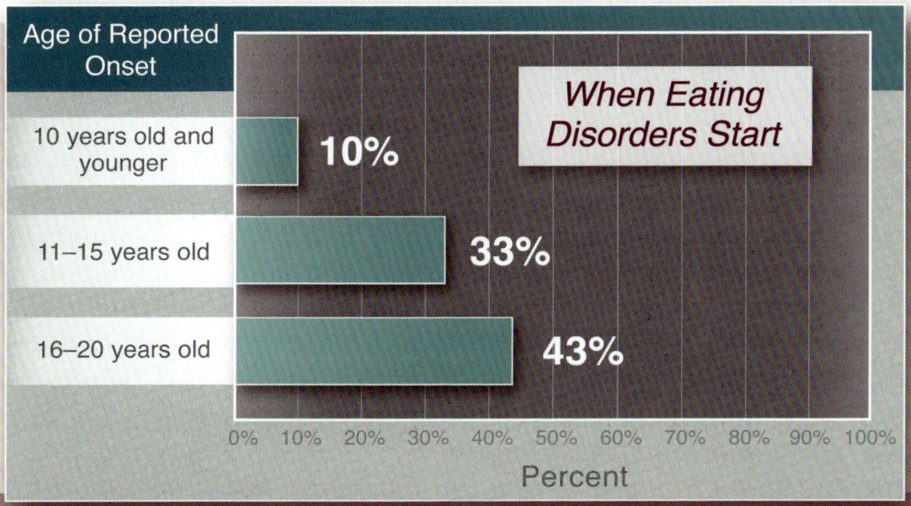

Source: "Identifying Eating Disorders in Children and Teens," The Emily Program, June 23, 2020. https://www.emilyprogram.com.

conditions in teens of both genders had worsened from 2010 to 2019. "More U.S. adolescents and young adults in the late 2010s, versus the mid-2000s, experienced serious psychological distress, major depression, or suicidal thoughts, and more attempted suicide,"[46] says Jean Twenge, a professor of psychology at San Diego State University.

Also, between 2010 and 2019 close to half of the young people with eating disorders had misused alcohol or illicit drugs five times more often than people in the general population. Even worse, some of the study participants had died. The NEDA reports that anorexics in their late teens were ten times more likely to die than their peers who did not have eating disorders.

The Perils of Distorted Body Image

It is only natural to wonder what has caused the major onslaught of eating disorders in teenagers both in the decades preceding the pandemic and after the COVID-19 virus appeared. In fact, many doctors and other experts say, it is essential that society comes to understand the causes in as much detail as possible in order to alleviate the widespread suffering associated with these insidious conditions. "The kids are not OK!" says Dr. Natalie D. Muth, director of the WELL healthy living clinic in Carlsbad, California. "It is on us to do everything we can to take steps and partner with our communities to safely return some normalcy to their lives."[47]

It stands to reason, the experts say, that some of the causes of eating disorders in teens will be the same as those that make adults develop those conditions. However, research conducted over the past half century has indicated that certain causes are peculiar to or much more common in adolescents. One factor that affects teens more often than grown-ups is a poor or distorted body image.

Distorted body image in an adolescent is largely based on the mistaken perception that he or she is unattractive, unintelligent, untalented, or worthless. That teenager tends to feel that he or she lacks the ability to meet the average social standards that his or her classmates take for granted. Therapists who specialize in eating disorders say that this young person tries to make up for what is supposedly lacking by finding some sort of coping mechanism. In simple terms, a coping mechanism is a method a person employs to try to compensate for or replace what is missing. Eating too much or too little food can be such a mechanism and in some cases can make the person feel a bit better in the short run.

In the long run, in contrast, eating more or less food than is natural or healthy for a given individual almost

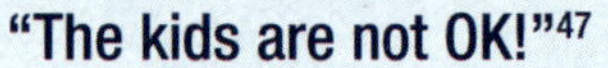

"The kids are not OK!"[47]

—Dr. Natalie D. Muth, director of the
WELL healthy living clinic in Carlsbad,
California

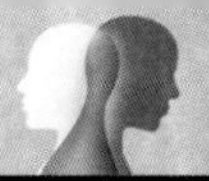

Ryan Raman, now in his thirties, tells about his experiences with poor body image when he was in his teens.

> For people like myself who struggle with body image issues, the way you view yourself is far more distorted than how other people view you. Having a negative perception of your body can promote feelings of anxiety, insecurity, and depression, and sometimes develop into an eating disorder. However, body image issues generally don't just appear out of thin air. They can be driven by factors like social media, bullying, and societal pressures. Growing up, I had a lot of insecurities. I was typically viewed as the chubby kid at school and had very few friends. Children are especially vulnerable to societal pressures and body image issues. . . . Because my weight was a factor I knew I could change. I had tried every new diet or trick I heard about to lose weight. However, the internet wasn't nearly as accessible as it is today, so I couldn't easily find healthy ways to lose weight. Instead, I believed that if I simply didn't eat food, I'd definitely lose weight.

Ryan Raman, "My Experience with Bulimia: A Dietician's Recovery Journey," Healthline, February 24, 2021. www.healthline.com.

invariably has various negative consequences. Only a few weeks or months of food misuse can in some young people bring on a full-fledged eating disorder. Making matters worse, it is not uncommon for adolescents to be unaware of what is happening to their body and emotional stability. According to Eating Disorders Victoria, an Australia-based support group for eating disorder sufferers, "Many [teens] with eating disorders do not realize they have a problem, or even if they do, they might not want to give up their behavior at first, because it is their mechanism for coping with an issue. Thus, they will go to extraordinary lengths to hide the signs of their behavior from people who care about them."[48]

Florence C., now in her twenties, was one of the teenagers who suffered from poor body image and paid the price by developing

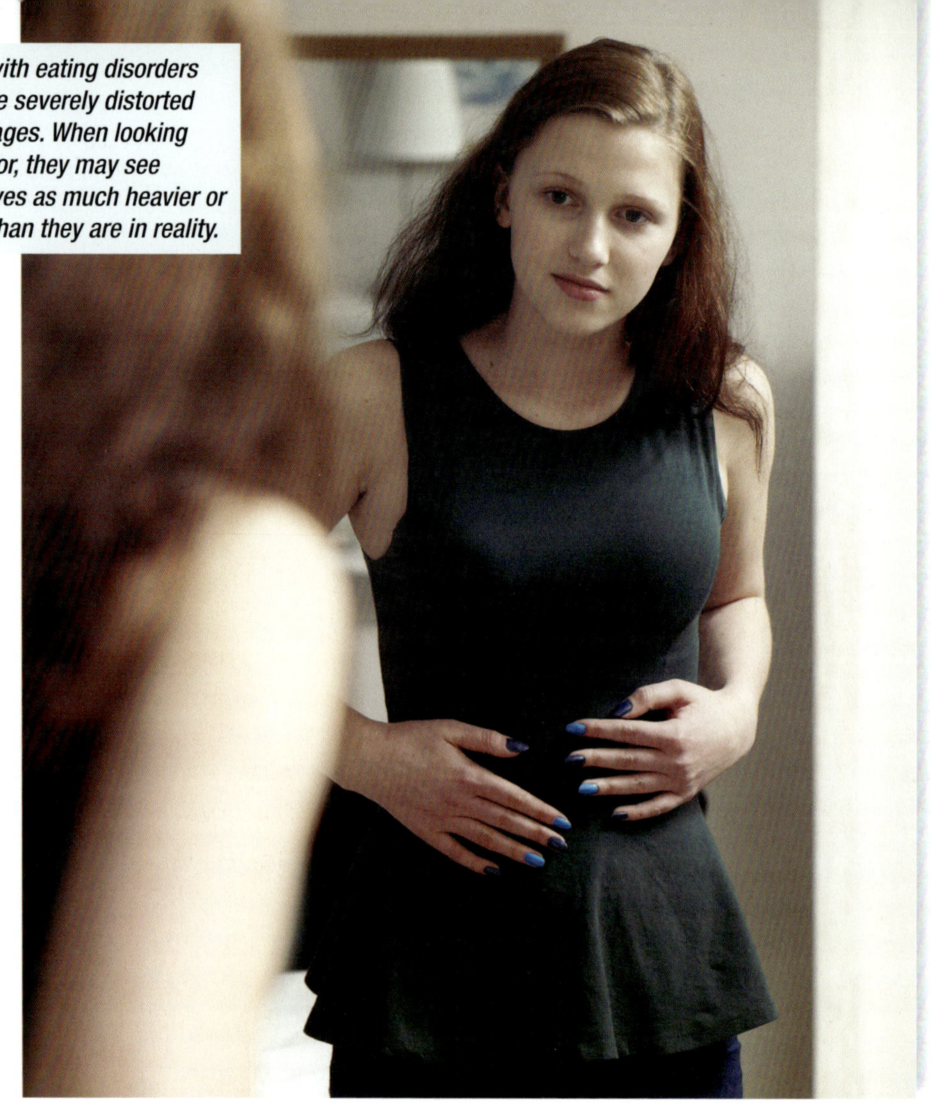

an eating disorder. "I firmly believed that I was fat," she recalls of her mental attitude during middle school. She realizes now that her weight was normal for her height. But at the time, she was convinced otherwise and for diverse reasons was unhappy with the way her life was going. She continues:

> It was after my freshman year of high school that I realized there was one thing that I could change, while providing a distraction from everything else in my life: my body. My weight loss was rapid; it disrupted everything in my life, and, at the time, it was a welcome distraction. . . . I thought

that losing weight was a way for me to make something change, until I realized that I had lost control of that too. I was hospitalized for the first time during my sophomore year, with a diagnosis of anorexia nervosa.[49]

Trying to Excel in Sports

Another factor that can help bring about an eating disorder in a young person's school years is a dedication to and yearning to do well in sports. Young female gymnasts, for example, are well known for shedding pounds to compete. According to the NEDA, this happens with up to 62 percent of school-age American female gymnasts.

Similar is major weight loss or gain by young male wrestlers, gymnasts, swimmers, divers, and even some football players. For a long time, most people did not recognize this problem in boys because eating disorders were incorrectly assumed to be conditions affecting only girls. Yet the reality, the NEDA points out, is that a whopping 33 percent of middle school and high school boys who play sports either develop an eating disorder or are at serious risk of doing so.

Missouri-born Joe, for instance, now in his seventies, blames his lifelong struggle with binge eating on his experiences as a high school wrestler. "The coach," he remembers,

> first had me gain ten or fifteen pounds so I could wrestle up a weight class. But later he told me to lose almost thirty pounds to fill a vacancy in a much lower weight class. To lose that weight and keep it off, I had to practically starve myself, and I learned later that the yo-yo weight gain and loss I repeatedly endured threw my metabolism way off, and I paid for it big-time in the decades that followed.[50]

Sean Canfield, a resident of Orlando, Florida, who is in his twenties, had a similar experience in his school years. At age

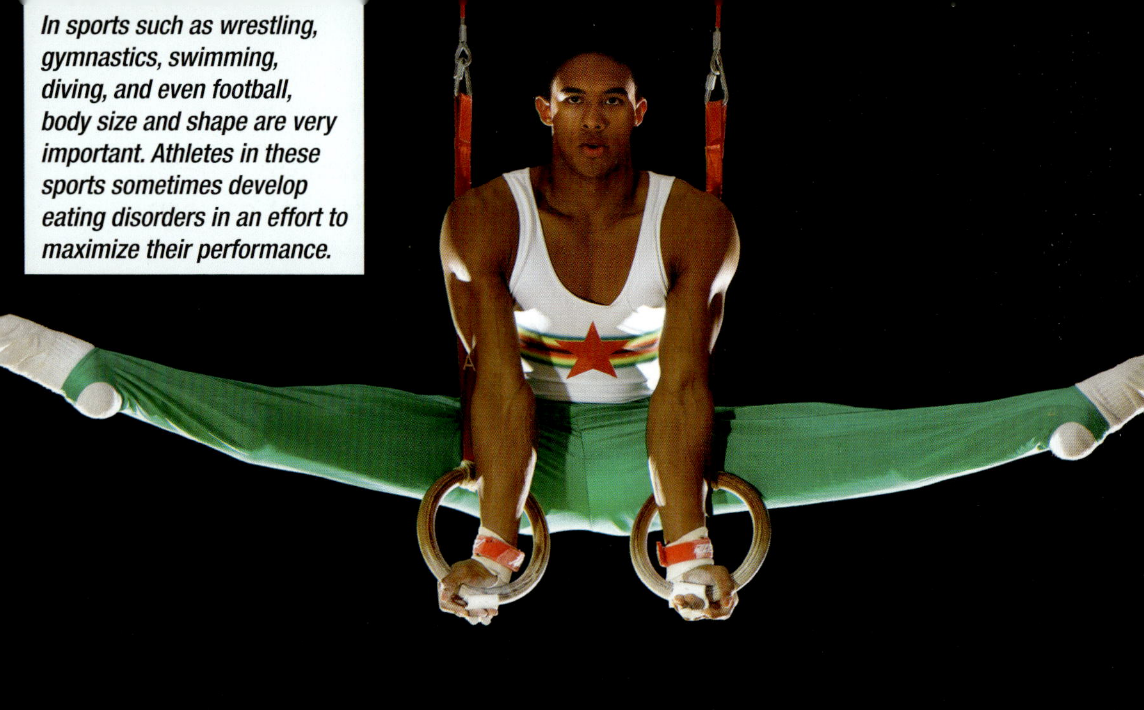

fourteen he developed anorexia, which rapidly worsened and led to his being hospitalized for heart damage caused by that potentially dangerous disorder. It all began, he recalls, when he tried out for his middle-school wrestling team. He remembers that he initially enjoyed the sport. Over time, however, he suffered several muscle injuries that forced the coach to bench him. Suddenly unhappy, he searched for ways to get back into competition. And assuming wrongly that his injuries had stemmed from excess pounds, he started losing weight. "I was trying to manipulate the only thing I really did have control over during that time," he says, "which was my diet. I became really focused on everything I ate, and it had to be perfect, and it couldn't have anything perceived 'unhealthy' about it. I was like, 'Fats, no, I can't touch that. Carbs, no.'" Later, after his grueling stint in the hospital, he says he learned that "when you are starved, your brain chemistry is all over the place. For me, instead of something that gives nourishment and happiness, food became a way of asserting control."[51] Now Canfield realizes he was out of control and almost died as a result.

Impact of Social Media and the Internet

The concept of control appears in a different context when it comes to the effects of social media and the internet on teenagers' eating habits and their development of eating disorders. Social media and other online sites have come to contribute to the incidence of eating disorders in adolescents in two ways. In the first, the people who host those sites often come to exert various degrees of control over the teens who make up their audience. Because members of that audience can be influenced by the hosts, the latter are sometimes called "influencers."

The primary reason that some of those influencers are a factor in the growth of eating disorders among adolescents is that many young people are eager for social acceptance and are willing to alter their look and identity to achieve that acceptance. As a result, teenagers may compare themselves to one or more influencers and try to imitate them. "Social media offers a constant way to compare yourself to others and to rely on superficial means of building self-esteem," explains Dr. Anne Marie O'Melia, chief medical officer of the Eating Recovery Center in Denver, Colorado. Such comparisons are typically bolstered by "how many 'likes' or comments you get on a post," she adds.

> "Social media offers a constant way to compare yourself to others and to rely on superficial means of building self-esteem."[52]
>
> —Dr. Anne Marie O'Melia of the Eating Recovery Center in Denver, Colorado

And unlike magazines or TV and movies, where even kids generally know there's a certain amount of professional make-up and editing happening, social media gives the impression that it's more "real," when it can be anything but. So young people are comparing themselves to an unrealistic and often impossible standard, which can lead to dangerous behaviors in an attempt to achieve something unachievable.[52]

The NEDA's Claire Mysko agrees. "We live in a culture where eating disorders thrive," she remarks, "because of the messages we're exposed to."[53] Many of those messages come from social media and other online sites, she says. And if the messages are that it is cool to be on the thin side and uncool to be overweight, then that can trigger the development of an eating disorder in an impressionable young person.

The other way that social media and the internet influence occurrences of eating disorders is by promoting them. Some people are shocked to learn about the existence of pro-ana, or pro-anorexia, websites. In the same vein, there are also pro-mia, or pro-bulimia, sites. Most of these sites preach—in direct contradiction to established scientific fact—that anorexia and bulimia are not disorders or illnesses. Rather, such sites claim, they are lifestyle choices or innocent trends or fads. Doctors, professional therapists, and hospitals caution that these websites are deceptive and potentially detrimental to the health of adolescents and anyone else who looks at them.

Moreover, some anorexics and bulimics abuse personal social media platforms such as Facebook, Twitter, and Instagram by using them to claim they are not ill. Instead, they insist, they have simply made personal choices to approach food in certain ways. Countering these bogus claims, however, are articles on the same platforms posted by teenage anorexics and bulimics who admit they are indeed sick. These individuals often tell their personal stories, including how they developed their disorder and where they have sought treatment.

Teens and Eating Disorders During the Pandemic

Social media and the internet contributed to the pervasiveness of eating disorders in teens before the pandemic, but their influence during that historic event likely worsened the problem. Young people, especially teens, are major users of social media and the various apps associated with them. Companies that keep track of online trends reported an increase of at least 20 percent in us-

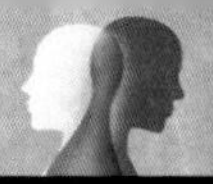

Benji Young, now an adult, is transgender. He recalls that when he was a teenager, a teacher covered eating disorders in school and the lesson stressed the age-old stereotypes about who suffers from such conditions. In a blog post on the NEDA website, he recounts his difficulties in coming to grips with his eating disorder.

> The paragraphs on anorexia and bulimia [in the book on health issues we were reading in class] described only the stereotype. Each paragraph described a middle-class or wealthy white female between 14 and 18 years old. . . . [The] book was missing male sufferers, transgender sufferers, African-American sufferers, sufferers living in poverty, overweight sufferers, [and so forth]. Each book was missing me. . . . Admitting I had an eating disorder was the hardest thing I ever had to do. I would later learn that I was not the only transgender young adult who struggled with an eating disorder. Eating disorders are not uncommon in the transgender community. Many people assume that all eating disorders are "typical," which makes those of us who don't fit the stereotype feel left out when we enter recovery. My disorder was never about my weight; it was about my gender identity.

Benji Young, "Ready to Accept," *Stories of Hope* (blog), National Eating Disorders Association, 2021. www.nationaleatingdisorders.org.

age of social media apps during the pandemic's first year—2020. In the United States a hefty portion of this usage was by adolescents. "In the context of the pandemic, teens are on social media more [than anyone else]," comments Alix Timko, a psychologist at Children's Hospital of Philadelphia. "That means they're potentially exposed to more content that could potentially trigger the development or maintenance of an eating disorder."[54]

Melissa Harrison, cofounder of the Center for Hope and Health, a treatment center for eating disorders in Ardmore, Pennsylvania, concurs. She says that she had many adolescent clients in 2020 who "learned ways to restrict their eating on TikTok."[55] Some, she adds, were as young as twelve.

Whether they used TikTok, Facebook, or some other social media platform, many teens focused their attention on the theme of weight—most often advocating that gaining weight was bad and losing it was good. Anne, a student in Massachusetts, commented in 2021 that "there was a general discourse on social media about not gaining weight during Covid or focusing on getting fit during Covid. So many people were equating self-improvement with weight loss or changing eating habits and it really affected me."[56]

Adolescents' use of social media during the pandemic might have aided the rise of eating disorders among teens, but so did some of the same core factors that prompted eating disorders in adults in that period. Isolation resulting from quarantining and social distancing took a particularly heavy toll. Moreover, such seclusion and the loneliness associated with it provided even more incentive for young people to turn to social media and the internet for support and comfort. Jillian Lampert, a staff member of the Emily Program, an organization that provides expert care to eating disorder sufferers, says she is not at all surprised that so many young people turned to social media. "Given the isolation that Covid brought," she states, "all of the messages on social media platforms were one of the main interactions that people had with the world."[57]

Another expert who was not surprised that young people's increased reliance on social media led to a rise in eating disorders during the COVID-19 outbreak is Lala T. Das, who works in a psychiatric illness emergency room. His main concern during the pandemic was that many of the teens diagnosed with those disorders did not know exactly where to turn for treatment. "In many of these cases," he says, "they or their family members recognized that something was wrong. In the setting of an overwhelmed system, however, they were unable to be linked to treatment."[58] However, he emphasizes that a wide array of treatments are available for teens with eating disorders and that their parents, teachers, and family doctors should help those young people seek them out.

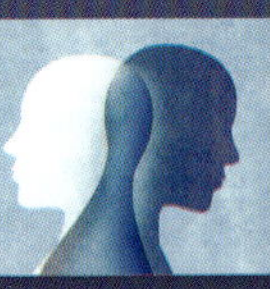

CHAPTER FOUR

Treating Eating Disorders

A young woman named Melissa says that when she was in her early twenties, her boyfriend told her she was getting too fat. She did not look very good when not wearing clothes, he added, and should start going to the gym. Melissa was understandably upset about what her boyfriend had said to her about her appearance. But she took some of what he said to heart. "I went on a diet to prove him wrong," she recalls. But unfortunately for her, "it spun out of control into an eating disorder."[59] She ate less and less, lost too much weight, and eventually even stopped feeling hungry most of the time.

At first Melissa did not discuss her problem with anyone. But after a while a close female friend noticed something was wrong and expressed concern. As a result, Melissa told her primary care physician about her dilemma. He sent her to a dietitian to help her reestablish healthy eating habits. The doctor also prescribed an antidepressant—medicine intended to increase her appetite, help her sleep, and generally make her feel better about herself.

In addition, because she seriously desired to get well, Melissa did a great deal of reading about eating disorders and became a minor expert on that topic. Partly as a result, she ended up working for an organization that provides care for people suffering from food-related disorders. In that capacity, she learned about the various treatments that exist for those sufferers.

Melissa also learned a somewhat disquieting fact that she managed to take in stride—namely, that she would likely never be fully cured of her disorder. "I don't think that [my eating disorder] will ever magically disappear," she says.

> I'm not cured of it; I simply manage it, day to day. It isn't a perfect process; it isn't like recovering from the flu, where one day you're sick, and then one day you're better. I see my eating disorder more as a disability now, a chronic condition, something that ebbs and flows, something that flares up. And I find that acknowledging that aspect of it—that recovery is less about perfection and more about management—allows me to have more compassion for myself as I move through this journey.[60]

A Combination of Approaches

Although eating disorders, like substance abuse disorders like alcoholism, cannot be cured completely, doctors and other experts point out that the situation is far from hopeless. Indeed, they say, these are conditions that can be controlled or managed. Thus, when people refer to themselves as "recovered anorexics" or "recovered bulimics," it means that they have learned to manage those conditions and keep them at bay from day to day, week to week, and year to year.

Aiding that management, as Melissa discovered, are a growing number of effective treatments for eating disorders. They fall into two general groups or types. One consists of trying to physically repair and heal a body that has undergone months or years of

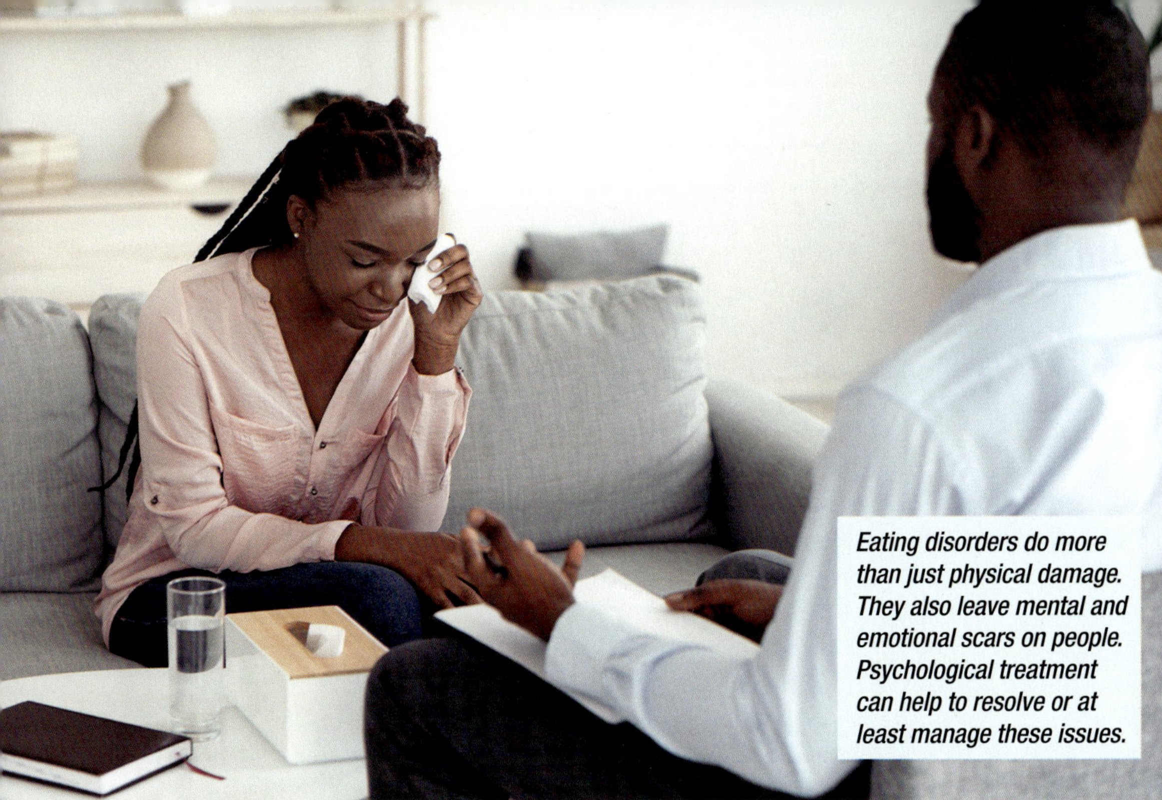

damage by fad diets, bingeing and purging, or starvation. The other common therapy consists of attempting to heal the mental and emotional scars the patient has obtained during her or his bout with such a disorder. This approach is most often referred to as psychological treatment.

These two general approaches are by no means mutually exclusive and are usually employed in combination. According to the NEDA, "Treating an eating disorder generally involves a combination of psychological and nutritional counseling, along with medical and psychiatric monitoring. Treatment must address the eating disorder symptoms and medical consequences, as well as psychological, biological, interpersonal, and cultural forces that contribute to or maintain the eating disorder."[61]

Hospitalization and Residential Care

Among the physical approaches to treating eating disorders, the one employed in the most extreme cases—in which a patient's life is on the line—is hospitalization. It can take two main forms,

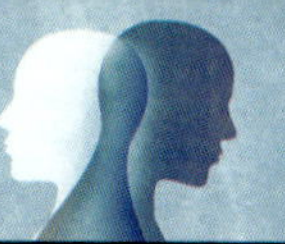

Although eating disorders can be treated, they cannot be totally cured. The main reason is that people with these conditions are addicted to food, or more precisely, to abusing food. Sufferers feel they cannot escape from or give up the source of their addiction. While an alcoholic or drug addict does not need these substances to live, every person requires food.

Binge eaters, anorexics, and bulimics cannot simply give up eating, since that would lead to starvation and death. Their treatment, then, cannot consist of refraining from indulging. Therefore, the only realistic choice is to learn to deal with food in ways that are as safe and healthy as possible. The fact that sufferers must continue to consume the "substance" they have long been abusing makes both recovery and safely managing the disorder extremely challenging goals.

inpatient care and outpatient care. In inpatient care, the patient stays in the hospital for as many days (or in the worst cases, weeks) as doctors feel is necessary. In contrast, outpatient care consists of the person with the eating disorder living at home and, if necessary, visiting the hospital once, twice, or more per week to undergo brief but rigorous testing.

As might be expected, the most extreme cases of eating disorders, in which anorexics have lost so much weight they are on the verge of death, require inpatient care. A website for the renowned Mayo Clinic states, "Severe or life-threatening physical health problems that occur with anorexia can be a medical emergency. In many cases, the most important goal of hospitalization is to stabilize acute medical symptoms through beginning the process of normalizing eating and weight."[62]

Once patients have been stabilized and their lives are no longer under imminent threat, various options are possible. Some individuals might be allowed to go home and periodically visit the hospital as an outpatient. Or under certain circumstances, home-care nurses might check in on the patient a few times a week.

At the same time, the patient might have periodic follow-up appointments with the attending doctor either at the hospital or at the doctor's office.

Still another option involving physical care is for the patient to spend some time in a residential facility. Most often such a place is a house-like building or group of buildings where multiple eating disorder patients live together for a few weeks or months and receive twenty-four-hour care. Such facilities feature strict daily schedules and structured living. But the benefit is that the patients—often called the "residents"—can concentrate on getting better while socializing with other people who are dealing with the same physical and emotional distress. The residents most often have meals together and spend time each day getting to know one another and sharing their personal stories.

Reactions to life in residential facilities for eating disorders vary. But many such residents experience it as did a teenager named Annabelle, whose parents placed her in such a facility for six weeks. At first, she felt lonely and out of place, but such negative reactions quickly faded. A couple of years later, she recalled:

It became the best thing I ever did. And it just changed my whole way of life, and yeah, I mean just the way I think, everything. I learned so much, and I made some amazingly good friends. And I think the most important thing, and the thing that helped me most was the staff because they were just so like caring and so amazing. And they really went out of their way to help. But it's not like . . . other places that I've been to [where] you just know that they're just doing it to get paid and they're like "Eeergh, when can we go home? I'm just sitting here watching you." But these people you know, a lot of them had first-hand experience of [what we were going though]. Some of them had [once had] eating disorders. And it . . . seemed to be their mission in life to get people well. And I really appreciate it.[63]

Medication and Counseling

Whether patients receive care for an eating disorder in a hospital, in a residential facility, or at home, often these people will receive some form of medication. Antidepressants are the most common kind of drug employed in treating these conditions, particularly binge eating and bulimia. According to clinical psychologist Lauren Muhlheim, the main goal in using them is to diminish or eliminate the incidents of bingeing and purging. "It is not yet known exactly why they work," she points out. What is more certain is that some antidepressants have "been shown to reduce binge eating, purging, and psychological symptoms such as the drive for thinness. This class of medications has demonstrated helpfulness with improving co-occurring symptoms of anxiety and depression."[64]

Anorexia is rarely treated in this manner. In fact, as late as 2021 the US Food and Drug Administration had not yet approved a specific medication for the treatment of anorexia. One problem with developing such a product is that testing its effectiveness and safety is extremely difficult. Muhlheim explains, "Treatment trials are considered difficult to conduct on patients with anorexia because these patients tend to be reluctant to take medication for fear of weight gain."[65]

Even when medications are used to treat eating disorders, typically they are employed in conjunction with psychological counseling, which the Mayo Clinic calls "the most important component of eating disorder treatment."[66] Sessions with a professional therapist who specializes in behavioral disorders, including ones related to food, may take place every day, a few times a week, or a few times a month, depending on the severity of the case and the needs of a given patient.

The chief aim of such counseling therapy is to help patients find a way to return to normal, healthy eating pat-

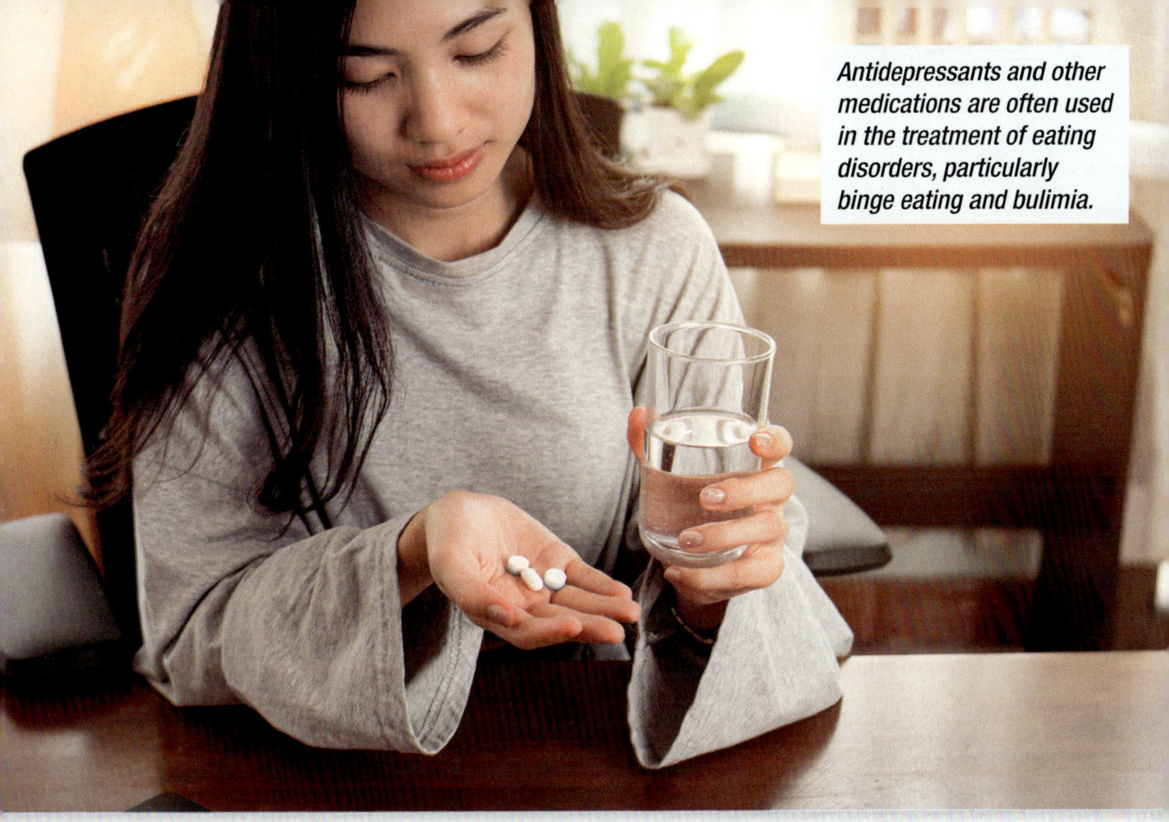

terns and a healthy weight. All involved hope that these patients will be able to maintain that weight, more or less, in the long term. To reach those goals, psychological counseling may utilize a handful of distinctive approaches. Among the most widely used is cognitive behavioral therapy (CBT), which focuses on managing or redirecting specific harmful behaviors and developing coping strategies. After talking about those behaviors over time with a therapist, patients can come to appreciate how their thought processes trigger their disordered eating habits.

Another kind of psychological therapy regularly employed in treating eating disorders is dialectical behavioral therapy (DBT). Using this method, therapists attempt to teach patients to refrain from coping with painful emotions by abusing food and, instead, to adopt healthier ways of dealing with such emotions. Binge eaters, for example, might learn effective ways of requesting the aid of family and friends for understanding and support. Or they might discover new ways of overcoming the powerful urge to overeat or eat too little.

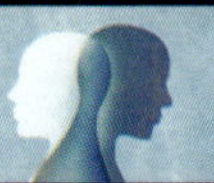

In addition to standard treatments for eating disorders, including medications, one-to-one sessions, and group therapy, the medical community is rapidly developing new approaches, including some that attempt to use genetic and other biologic information to predict susceptibility to eating disorders. As Angela Guarda, a spokesperson for the American Psychiatric Association, summarizes it:

> Research on eating disorders is progressing rapidly. It is now clear that eating disorders are biologically based illnesses, not simple lifestyle choices. Recent genetic work has focused on identifying genes that increase risk for an eating disorder and on [gene-related] interactions that may contribute to the onset of an eating disorder. Brain imaging research is examining altered decision making around food choice and reward learning in individuals with eating disorders. Other lines of research focus on improving insight into how starvation, exercise and binge purge behaviors [interfere with] brain reward circuits and gut-brain signaling, and whether these changes contribute to the driven, compulsive nature of eating and weight control behaviors. This is exciting work that holds promise for developing novel treatments in the coming years.

Angela Guarda, "Expert Q + A: Eating Disorders," American Psychiatric Association, 2020. www.psychiatry.org.

Ryan Raman underwent both CBT and DBT with his therapist and says that these methods greatly helped him learn to control and live with his bulimia. "I decided to seek help," he recalls,

and work alongside a therapist and healthcare professional to change my body perception and build a healthier relationship with food. Together, we were able to identify the thought patterns and beliefs that contributed to my bulimia. We worked on finding ways to change my perception of them and developed a maintenance plan to help prevent a relapse in the future. Although the process took a while, I'm thankful for the support from my healthcare provider, therapist, and friends, who were alongside me throughout the journey. They provided me with the safe space I needed to face this challenge head-on.[67]

Group and Nutritional Therapy

The discussions that Raman had with his counselor are generally referred to as one-to-one sessions. Most doctors who treat eating disorders recommend that patients eventually move on to a collective form of counseling called group therapy. The reason is that group therapy often produces benefits for patients that would be a good deal harder to accomplish in a one-to-one setting. According to the experts at the UK-based health care organization Priory:

> The use of group methods in psychotherapy rests on the central idea that exposure to one's own problems and pain as they are experienced in the lives of the others facing you can bring about change of an unforeseen kind with far-reaching consequences. . . . [Group sessions] can relieve emotional pain, untie isolation, resolve distress, provide healing and bring about changes to a person's thoughts and emotions as well as their personal relations. . . . Working in a group setting, making connections and sharing experiences of their own can provide people with the crucial opportunity to be heard and seen, helping them to understand that they are not alone.[68]

Doctors and other experts also highly recommend nutritional therapy, which they say can be an effective supplement to psychological counseling. At the most basic level, eating disorders stem from the abuse of food, so it makes sense for experts on food and nutrition to bring their knowledge and experience into the treatment arena.

Coordinating with a doctor, a nutritional therapist zeros in on deficiencies or irregularities in patients' diets. To do that, usually the therapist looks at patients' eating history and determines their favorite foods. The therapist also finds out whether the patients have repeatedly been on fad reducing diets, which is often the case. Have these individuals frequently gained weight, lost it, and gained it again? By asking such questions, the nutritional therapist puts together a detailed picture of each patient's former eating habits; then the therapist uses that information to make recommendations about changing those habits. When appropriate, the therapist suggests a generalized meal plan, as well as points out which foods to avoid because they can be triggers for disordered eating.

Other Kinds of Therapy

Nutritional therapy is basic and straightforward in its approach, as well as pretty much necessary and unavoidable in the treatment process. Meanwhile, over the years therapists have devised a few more creative approaches that can be used as supplements in treating eating disorders. In one, usually called dance movement therapy (or more simply dance therapy), patients express feelings and emotions through a series of dance steps and body movements. The core concept is for the patients to utilize nonverbal means of conveying those feelings and emotions. The therapist watches and interprets specific movements in ways that at least partially reveal each patient's state of mind.

Similarly, so-called art therapy attempts to get patients to express their innermost feelings, both negative and positive. Art therapy itself first appeared in the mid-twentieth century and was initially employed to help patients suffering from serious mental disorders. Later, in the century's last two decades, a few therapists saw its potential for treating eating disorders. In a typical art therapy session, patients draw, paint, sculpt, or delve into some other form of artistic medium. The counselor usually requests that patients produce images or objects that capture their innermost feelings or thoughts. Then patients and therapist discuss the meaning of the artwork and how it might affect any feelings, especially those relating to the specific eating disorders.

Other types of creative therapy for eating disorders include equine therapy, which exploits the relationship between a patient and a horse; and canine therapy, which does the same thing with one or more dogs. These and other approaches that involve animals, Eating Disorder Hope explains, take advantage of the fact that real emotional bonds can grow between humans and animals and that such situations can "allow for emotional healing to occur. Activities that might be involved are care for and grooming of the animal and basic exercises guided by an [animal] specialist. Men or women who use [such animal-based] therapy during treatment might have increased self-esteem and body image, particularly as the care for an animal has been shown to be an empowering experience."[69]

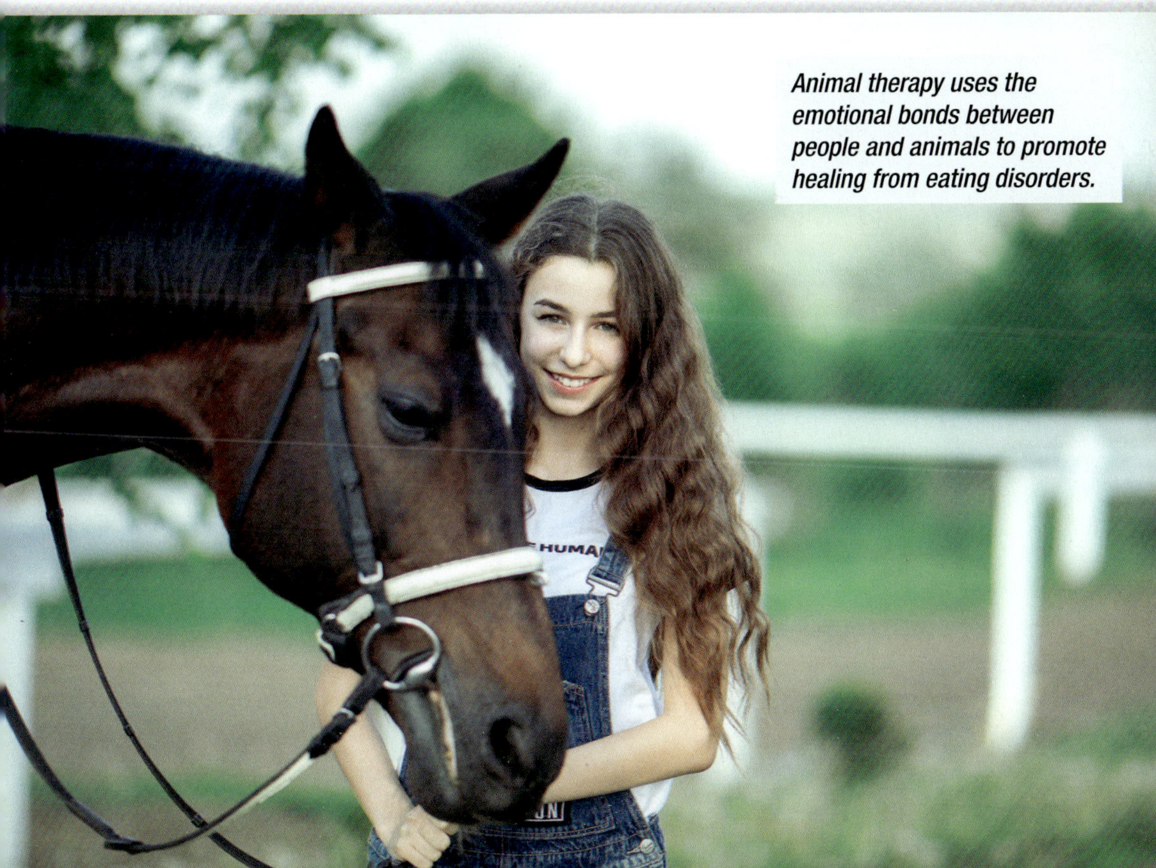

Animal therapy uses the emotional bonds between people and animals to promote healing from eating disorders.

Whichever types of therapy end up being used for a given patient, doctors, therapists, and successful patients alike stress that seeking treatment for one's eating disorder is essential. Unfortunately, most eating disorders tend to get worse if left untreated. For comfort, peace of mind, and ultimately personal happiness, a person afflicted with such a disorder should start treatment as soon as possible. As Raman puts it:

> Just starting the conversation with someone you trust can make you feel as if you've had a massive weight lifted off of your shoulders. Eating disorders are complicated, and there's no quick fix. Instead, they often require working with various health professionals like doctors, dietitians, and therapists, all of whom have your best interest at heart. While seeking help may seem daunting at first, it's important to know that you're not alone, and the road to recovery starts with one little step.[70]

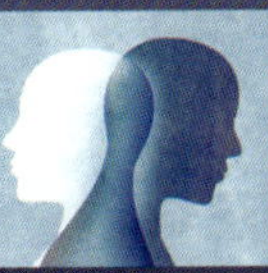

Introduction: A Significant Social and Medical Hazard

1. Quoted in Kelty Mental Health Resource Centre, "Sara's Story," 2021. https://keltyeatingdisorders.ca.
2. Quoted in Kelty Mental Health Resource Centre, "Sara's Story."
3. Quoted in Kelty Mental Health Resource Centre, "Sara's Story."
4. Quoted in Vanessa Caceres, "Eating Disorder Statistics," *U.S. News & World Report*, February 14, 2020. https://health.usnews.com.
5. Quoted in Eric Graber, "Eating Disorders on the Rise," American Society for Nutrition, February 22, 2021. https://nutrition.org.
6. Kathy Katella, "Eating Disorders on the Rise in Pandemic," Yale Medicine, June 15, 2021. www.yalemedicine.org.
7. Mayo Clinic, "Eating Disorders," February 22, 2018. www.mayoclinic.org.
8. Quoted in Chris Willman, "Taylor Swift Opens Up About Overcoming Struggle with Eating Disorder," *Variety*, January 23, 2020. https://variety.com.

Chapter One: The Big Three Eating Disorders

9. Ben, "Young, Professional, Male—and Living with an Eating Disorder," Eating Disorders Victoria, 2019. www.eatingdisorders.org.au.
10. Ben, "Young, Professional, Male—and Living with an Eating Disorder."
11. National Eating Disorders Association, "What Are Eating Disorders," 2021. www.nationaleatingdisorders.org.
12. Rachel Goodman, "The Dos and Don'ts to Stop Binge Eating," Rachel Good Nutrition, 2019. https://rachelgoodnutrition.com.
13. Quoted in MEDA, "Jack's Story," 2021. www.medainc.org.
14. Quoted in MEDA, "Jack's Story."
15. Eating Disorder Hope, "What Is Bulimia: Symptoms, Complications and Causes," 2021. www.eatingdisorderhope.com.

16. National Institute of Mental Health, "Eating Disorders," 2021. www
.nimh.nih.gov.
17. Amanda Goheen, "Recovery Is a Journey, Not a Destination," *Stories of Hope* (blog), National Eating Disorders Association, 2021.
www.nationaleatingdisorders.org.
18. Julie Saunders, "Road to Recovery," *Stories of Hope* (blog), National Eating Disorders Association, 2021. www.nationaleating
disorders.org.
19. *Psychology Today*, "What Are Eating Disorders?," 2021. www.psy
chologytoday.com.
20. *Psychology Today*, "What Are Eating Disorders?"
21. Ben, "Young, Professional, Male—and Living with an Eating Disorder."
22. Seth Bland, "'You Don't Have to Live like This,'" *Stories of Hope* (blog), National Eating Disorders Association, 2021. www.national
eatingdisorders.org.
23. Saunders, "Road to Recovery."
24. Eating Disorder Hope, "Diet Fads and Eating Disorders," 2021. www.eatingdisorderhope.com.
25. Ashley Marcin, "Bulimia Took a Decade from My Life. Don't Make My Mistake," Healthline, April 18, 2019. www.healthline.com.

Chapter Two: The COVID-19 Pandemic and the Rise in Eating Disorders

26. Quoted in Mollie Ames, "Patterns During the Pandemic: How Eating Disorders Have Affected College Students During COVID-19," Mary Christie Institute, July 14, 2021. https://marychristieinstitute.org.
27. Quoted in Ames, "Patterns During the Pandemic."
28. Quoted in Ishani Chettri and Michelle Vassilev, "Social Media, Isolation Exacerbated Eating Disorders During Pandemic, Students Say," *GW Hatchet* (Washington, DC), August 23, 2021. www.gw
hatchet.com.
29. Julia F. Taylor and Sara Groff Stephens, "The COVID-19 Pandemic Increased Eating Disorders Among Young People—but the Signs Aren't What Parents Might Expect," The Conversation, November 2, 2021. https://theconversation.com.
30. Quoted in Iris Goldsztajn, "The Second Pandemic: Eating Disorders Are Surging, and They Won't Stop When COVID Does," *InStyle*, February 25, 2021. www.instyle.com.
31. Quoted in Ames, "Patterns During the Pandemic."
32. Dawn Branley-Bell and Catherine V. Talbot, "Exploring the Impact of the COVID-19 Pandemic and UK Lockdown on Individuals with Experience of Eating Disorders," *Journal of Eating Disorders*, August 2020. https://jeatdisord.biomedcentral.com/articles/10.1186
/s40337-020-00319-y.
33. Quoted in Ezgi Toper, "Tiktok, Covid Bubbles and Body Image: Why Eating Disorders Are on the Rise," TRT World, April 29, 2021. www
.trtworld.com.

34. Quoted in Toper, "Tiktok, Covid Bubbles and Body Image."
35. Branley-Bell and Talbot, "Exploring the Impact of the COVID-19 Pandemic and UK Lockdown on Individuals with Experience of Eating Disorders."
36. Quoted in Branley-Bell and Talbot, "Exploring the Impact of the COVID-19 Pandemic and UK Lockdown on Individuals with Experience of Eating Disorders."
37. Quoted in Branley-Bell and Talbot, "Exploring the Impact of the COVID-19 Pandemic and UK Lockdown on Individuals with Experience of Eating Disorders."
38. Quoted in Branley-Bell and Talbot, "Exploring the Impact of the COVID-19 Pandemic and UK Lockdown on Individuals with Experience of Eating Disorders."
39. Taylor and Stephens, "The COVID-19 Pandemic Increased Eating Disorders Among Young People—but the Signs Aren't What Parents Might Expect."
40. Quoted in Michelle Tauber, "Eating Disorders Surge in Boys and Young Men: What Parents Need to Know," *People*, August 11, 2021. https://people.com.
41. Quoted in Naveen Kumar, "Eating Disorders in Men Are Not Talked About Enough—and They're on the Rise," Healthline, November 23, 2021. www.healthline.com.
42. National Eating Disorders Association, "Eating Disorders in LGBTQ+ Populations," 2021. www.nationaleatingdisorders.org.
43. Jennifer Tabler et al., "Perceived Weight Gain and Eating Disorder Symptoms Among LGBTQ Adults During the COVID-19 Pandemic: A Convergent Mixed-Method Study," *Journal of Eating Disorders*, September 16, 2021. www.ncbi.nlm.nih.gov.
44. Branley-Bell and Talbot, "Exploring the Impact of the COVID-19 Pandemic and UK Lockdown on Individuals with Experience of Eating Disorders."

Chapter Three: Eating Disorders in Teens

45. Quoted in Carly Menker, "Pandemic Fuels Rise in Eating Disorders Among Adolescents," American Academy of Pediatrics, *AAP News*, June 1, 2021. https://publications.aap.org.
46. Quoted in American Psychological Association, "Mental Health Issues Increased Significantly in Young Adults over Last Decade," March 14, 2019. www.apa.org.
47. Quoted in Menker, "Pandemic Fuels Rise in Eating Disorders Among Adolescents."
48. Eating Disorders Victoria, "Eating Disorders Explained," 2019. www.eatingdisorders.org.au.

49. Florence C., "A Project in the Making," *Stories of Hope* (blog), National Eating Disorders Association, 2021. www.nationaleating disorders.org.
50. Joe, personal interview with the author, December 2, 2021.
51. Quoted in Tauber, "Eating Disorders Surge in Boys and Young Men."
52. Quoted in Menker, "Pandemic Fuels Rise in Eating Disorders Among Adolescents."
53. Quoted in Marceia Rojas, "Social Media Helps Fuel Some Eating Disorders," *USA Today*, June 1, 2014. www.usatoday.com.
54. Quoted in Toper, "Tiktok, Covid Bubbles and Body Image."
55. Quoted in Toper, "Tiktok, Covid Bubbles and Body Image."
56. Quoted in William A. Haseltine, "How the Pandemic Is Fueling Eating Disorders in Young People," *Forbes*, August 27, 2021. www .forbes.com.
57. Quoted in Haseltine, "How the Pandemic Is Fueling Eating Disorders in Young People."
58. Lala T. Das, "Eating Disorders Are Exploding, Hurting Adolescents Who Have Trouble Finding Care," *Washington Post*, September 3, 2021. www.washingtonpost.com.

Chapter Four: Treating Eating Disorders

59. Quoted in Brittany Risher, "10 People Who Have Dealt with Eating Disorders Share What Recovery Looks like for Them," *Self*, November 16, 2018. www.self.com.
60. Quoted in Risher, "10 People Who Have Dealt with Eating Disorders Share What Recovery Looks like for Them."
61. National Eating Disorders Association, "What to Expect from Treatment," 2021. www.nationaleatingdisorders.org.
62. Mayo Clinic, "Eating Disorder Treatment: Know Your Options," July 14, 2017. www.mayoclinic.org.
63. Healthtalk, "Eating Disorders (Young People): Staying in Hospital," 2019. https://healthtalk.org.
64. Lauren Muhlheim, "Medications Used to Treat Eating Disorders," Verywell Mind, July 17, 2020. www.verywellmind.com.
65. Muhlheim, "Medications Used to Treat Eating Disorders."
66. Mayo Clinic, "Eating Disorder Treatment."
67. Ryan Raman, "My Experience with Bulimia: A Dietician's Recovery Journey," Healthline, February 24, 2021. www.healthline.com.
68. Priory, "How Group Therapy Can Help Those with Eating Disorders," 2021. www.priorygroup.com.
69. Eating Disorder Hope, "Types of Eating Disorder Treatment & Therapy," 2021. www.eatingdisorderhope.com.
70. Raman, "My Experience with Bulimia."

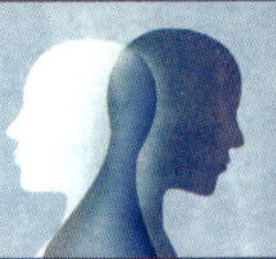

Emily Program
www.emilyprogram.com
Founded in 1993, the Emily Program is a nationally recognized treatment program. Its website provides information about eating disorders, links to experts and clinics treating these disorders, and psychological support for sufferers of all ages. It also includes a section for families that teens will benefit from.

Help with Eating Disorders, American Psychiatric Association (APA)
www.psychiatry.org/patients-families/eating-disorders
The APA's main website on eating disorders contains numerous links to information not only about eating disorders but also about often related problems that can affect teens and other young people, including substance abuse and obsessive-compulsive disorder.

National Association of Anorexia Nervosa and Associated Disorders (ANAD)
www.anad.org
ANAD focuses on the prevention of eating disorders and educates and helps people who need to find treatment and support. Teens will benefit directly from ANAD's twenty-four-hour help line, as well as school outreach programs for school-age youth and peer support groups for people of various ages.

National Eating Disorder Information Centre (NEDIC)
https://nedic.ca
NEDIC is the primary support organization for people with eating disorders in Canada. The website directs teens and others with these disorders to a free help line or an instant chat feature. In addition, the site contains blogs written by people affected by eating disorders.

National Eating Disorders Association (NEDA)
www.nationaleatingdisorders.org
The NEDA is recognized as the United States' foremost eating disorders support group. The website provides access to twenty-four-hour help for people of all ages who suffer from eating disorders. The website also addresses the needs of LGBTQ people who have these harmful disorders.

National Institute of Mental Health (NIMH)
www.nimh.nih.gov
Part of the National Institutes of Health, the NIMH provides information about the causes, prevention, treatment, and recovery from eating disorders. Teens will benefit from an online chat feature, along with links to social media versions of the NIMH information center.

National Suicide Prevention Lifeline
https://suicidepreventionlifeline.org
1 (800) 273-8255
The National Suicide Prevention Lifeline is a national network of local crisis centers. It operates around the clock and provides free and confidential support for people experiencing a suicidal crisis or emotional distress.

Books

Bethany Brian, *Dealing with Eating Disorders*. San Diego, CA: ReferencePoint, 2020.

Kevin Hayes, *Eating Disorders Information for Teens*. Detroit, MI: Omnigraphics, 2021.

Katie Sharp, *Pandemic Aftereffects: The Surge in Teen Eating Disorders*. San Diego, CA: ReferencePoint, 2023.

Rosalyn Sheehy and Simona Donzelli, *Food Fight Club: Rules to Beat Bulimia*. Virginia Beach, VA: Koehler, 2021.

Mary Tantillo, *Multifamily Therapy Group for Young Adults with Anorexia Nervosa*. London: Routledge, 2020.

Kristin Thiel, *Dealing with Eating Disorders*. New York: Cavendish Square, 2019.

Internet Sources

Behavioral Nutrition, "The Prevalence of Eating Disorders in America," 2018. https://behavioralnutrition.org.

Vanessa Caceres, "Eating Disorder Statistics," *U.S. News & World Report*, February 14, 2020. https://health.usnews.com.

Julie Jargon, "Boys Have Eating Disorders, Too. Doctors Think Social Media Is Making It Worse," *Wall Street Journal*, November 13, 2021. www.wsj.com.

JED Foundation, "Understanding Food and Body Image Struggles." https://jedfoundation.org.

Mayo Clinic, "Binge-Eating Disorder," May 5, 2018. www.mayoclinic.org.

Carly Menker, "Pandemic Fuels Rise in Eating Disorders Among Adolescents," American Academy of Pediatrics, *AAP News*, June 1, 2021. https://publications.aap.org.

National Eating Disorders Association, "Bulimia Nervosa," 2021. www.nationaleatingdisorders.org.

National Eating Disorders Association, "Eating Disorders in LGBTQ+ Populations," 2021. www.nationaleatingdisorders.org.

National Eating Disorders Association, "Orthorexia," 2021. www.nationaleatingdisorders.org.

Psychology Today, "Anorexia Nervosa," 2021. www.psychologytoday.com.

Psychology Today, "What Are Eating Disorders?," 2021. www.psychologytoday.com.

SingleCare Team, "Eating Disorder Statistics 2021," *The Checkup* (blog), SingleCare, January 21, 2021. www.singlecare.com.

Peter Suciu, "Social Media Can Increase Risk of Eating Disorders and Negative Body Image," *Forbes*, February 24, 2021. www.forbes.com.

Julia F. Taylor and Sara Groff Stephens, "The COVID-19 Pandemic Increased Eating Disorders Among Young People—but the Signs Aren't What Parents Might Expect," The Conversation, November 2, 2021. https://theconversation.com.

Ezgi Toper, "Tiktok, Covid Bubbles and Body Image: Why Eating Disorders Are on the Rise," TRT World, April 29, 2021. www.trtworld.com.

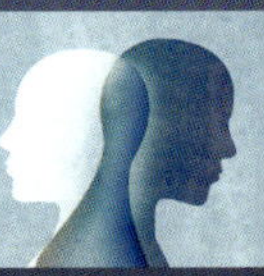